A WOMAN DOCTOR'S GUIDE TO OSTEOPOROSIS

A WOMAN DOCTOR'S GUIDE TO OSTEOPOROSIS

Essential Facts and Up-to-the-Minute
Information on the Prevention,
Treatment, and Reversal of Bone Loss

By

Yvonne R. Sherrer, M.D.

with

Robin K. Levinson

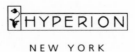

NEW YORK

LIBRARY OF CONGRESS CATALOGING-IN-PUBLICATION DATA

Sherrer, Yvonne R.
    A woman doctor's guide to osteoporosis : essential facts and up-to-the-minute information on the prevention, treatment, and reversal of bone loss / Yvonne R. Sherrer, with Robin K. Levinson; illustrations by Mona Mark.
        p.   cm.
    Includes index.
    ISBN 0-7868-8045-7
    1. Osteoporosis—Popular works.   2. Women—Diseases.
I. Levinson, Robin K.   II. Title.
RC931.073S54   1995
616.7′16—dc20   94-15044
                                                                    CIP

FIRST EDITION

10 9 8 7 6 5 4 3 2 1

I dedicate this book to my parents, George and Roberta Smallwood, and to my loving family, Chris, Salome, Joy, and Nathan.

—Dr. Yvonne R. Smallwood Sherrer

I dedicate this book to my late grandmother, Mamie Michaels.

—Robin K. Levinson

CONTENTS

LIST OF
ILLUSTRATIONS

INTRODUCTION

Do you shudder at the thought of looking like the "little old lady from Pasadena"—a frail woman with a hump in her back, constant pain, and a walking cane? Are you afraid of breaking a hip and winding up in a nursing home? For an estimated 20 million women with osteoporosis in the United States, those fears are justified. Instead of supporting and protecting them as healthy skeletons should, their skeletons have thinned out to the point where their bones can break under the slightest trauma or while they are doing mundane tasks. Depending on the site of the fracture, the break can result in chronic pain, loss of height, damaged self-esteem, disfigurement, and, in extreme cases, loss of independence and even death.

Osteoporosis has reached epidemic proportions in this country and around the world. Its growing scope and financial burden have prompted a wave of scientific investigations into its causes, prevention, and treatments. No definitive "cure" has been discovered, but researchers have garnered a wealth of knowledge that translates into a bevy of hormonal and medicinal treatments and diet and exercise recommendations that can often prevent, mitigate, or even reverse the potentially devastating consequences of osteoporosis.

The fact that you're reading this book means you've been diagnosed with osteoporosis, know someone suffering with the condition, or want to learn how to prevent it or help someone you love keep her bones healthy and strong. This book can help on all counts.

In Part I, you will learn about the fascinating processes that take place in bone tissue at the microscopic level. You will learn why, in some people, bones become "porous," and in others, they remain denser and stronger. You will get tips on finding a doctor and other health-care professionals to treat the condition. And you will see how physicians diagnose osteoporosis and determine who is at risk.

In Part II, you will get the latest information on osteoporosis treatments and preventions. The roles played by estrogen, calcium and other nutritional factors as well as exercise will be discussed in detail. You will learn what girls and younger women can do to prevent osteoporosis in their later years. And you will meet three women who have been assaulted by the disorder sometimes called "the silent thief."

PART I
OSTEOPOROSIS: THE SILENT EPIDEMIC

CHAPTER 1

WHAT IS OSTEOPOROSIS?

Since the time of Hippocrates, it has been evident that thinning bones are a natural consequence of aging. From Hippocrates' time in the fifth century B.C. until the beginning of the twentieth century, most people died long before their bones thinned to the point of causing fractures. Not true today. Life expectancy has grown markedly in the latter half of the twentieth century, as has the population. In 1991, one in three American women was 50 or older. The baby-boom generation will begin to enter their retirement years soon after the turn of the century. The average woman lives some thirty years after menopause. Thanks in part to medical advances and the emphasis on exercise and healthy diets, vast numbers of boomers can expect to reach their eighties, nineties, or beyond. If present-day trends continue unabated, osteoporosis threatens to be one of the biggest public-health menaces of modern times.

Osteoporosis, literally "porous bones," is not a disease, per se. It's the end result of an insidious, symptomless process that begins around age 35 or 40 but that may not be discovered until twenty or thirty years later when bones begin to break. Osteoporosis is one of the leading causes of disability in the United States and the most common cause of hip fracture. Hip fracture can lead to disability, loss of independence, and, in rare cases, death.

A woman's problem

Although men can be affected, osteoporosis is primarily an older woman's problem. Eighty percent of the more than 25 million Americans with osteoporosis are female, partly because women generally have smaller bones and live longer than men. Excessive bone loss affects more than half of all women over 65, and osteoporosis has been detected in as many as 90 percent of women over age 75. The U.S. Census Bureau projects that the number of Americans age 85 and older—those at highest risk for osteoporosis—will triple by 2012.

One in three postmenopausal white women will suffer at least one osteoporosis-induced fracture in her lifetime, experts say. Each year another 1.5 million postmenopausal women develop brittle bones due to osteoporosis. According to government data, of the 2 million or so bone fractures that occur in the United States annually, 1.3 million are caused by osteoporosis. Of those 1.3 million fractures, 300,000 are osteoporotic fractures of the hip bone. By 2020, the number of hip fractures is projected to reach 350,000 and by 2040, to exceed 500,000. Primarily through complications stemming from hip fractures, osteoporosis kills an estimated 50,000 Americans annually, most of them women.

Economic burden

In addition to the physical and emotional tolls on its victims, osteoporosis exacts an enormous financial burden on society: $10 billion to $18 billion is spent on osteoporosis medical and nursing care annually, according to the National Osteoporosis Foundation (NOF), a Washington, D.C.–based nonprofit organization devoted to reducing the prevalence of osteoporosis. It is further estimated that osteoporosis costs more than $7 billion a year in lost wages. If osteoporosis and health-care inflation grow unchecked, osteoporosis costs will mushroom to more than $60 billion by 2020, the NOF warns. With aggressive screening and prevention programs, however, some experts believe that osteoporosis can go the way of measles in this country. "Even a small percent reduction in the incidence of hip fractures could save several thousand lives and several millions of dollars each year," states the 1985 Johns Hopkins University publication *Epidemiologic Reviews*.

WHAT CAUSES OSTEOPOROSIS?

Bone tissue is continually removed and replaced by specialized cells. The reasons behind this biological process will be discussed in Chapter 2. During childhood and into young adulthood, more bone is made than is taken away. This so-called bone "remodeling" process reaches an equilibrium by age 35 to 40, after which the skeleton begins to lose more tissue than it creates. For reasons not clearly understood, the imbalance grows more severe as people age. The imbalance has been associated with the slow withdrawal of sex hormones as people get older. In women, the female sex hormone, estrogen, diminishes as a woman approaches the age of menopause. For several years after menopause, bone loss accelerates. In women who failed to build up enough bone density earlier in life, this bone loss can eventually weaken the skeleton to the point where it can fracture under the minor stresses of everyday activities, such as cooking, getting out of a car, opening a window, making a bed, or getting a hug. Fractures of the vertebra, known as "crush" or "compression" fractures, can also happen spontaneously under the pressure of gravity alone.

Sarah Steele (not her real name), 62, suffered her first crushed vertebra in 1988 during a sneeze. "I did a foolish thing," the Boca Raton, Florida, jewelry maker says. "I held my nose and covered my mouth and the sneeze sort of exploded inside of me. I actually heard the crack in my back." Since then Sarah has suffered three more crushed vertebrae: one while powdering her nose, one while bending over, and one she was unaware of until her back was X-rayed. Sarah, who had always had good posture, has lost two inches of height as a result of osteoporosis. Her upper back is beginning to bow.

Even though most of Sarah's fractures happened suddenly, her bones had been losing density for years, perhaps decades. As mentioned earlier, osteoporosis is the end result of years of thinning bones, just as a heart attack is the end result of years of damaged, clogged arteries. When bones are losing density but have not reached what's known as the "fracture zone," the condition is called osteopenia. One study in Michigan found that more than half the women over age 45 showed evidence of osteopenia on spinal X-rays. Having osteopenia doesn't necessarily mean that you will develop osteoporosis, especially if you take steps to preserve existing bone or build bone density back up.

If your bone mass is low enough, you can be diagnosed with osteoporosis even if you've never had a fracture. Such a diagnosis means you are at extremely high risk for fractures unless you do something to protect yourself.

Bone-density-measuring technology can diagnose both osteoporosis and osteopenia. By getting a diagnosis and treatment early, you may be able to stay out of the fracture zone. If you are already in the fracture zone, keeping your home free of hazards and practicing proper body mechanics can reduce your risk of breaking a bone.

Types of osteoporosis

There are two general classifications and three recognized types of osteoporosis, plus a fourth type that is not formally labeled in the medical literature. When osteoporosis stems from menopause or aging, the classification is "primary osteoporosis." When it results from another disease, a medication, or a surgical procedure, it is classified as "secondary osteoporosis." Your physician should determine your classification and type of osteoporosis before prescribing treatment. If you have a disease known to cause bone loss or are taking a medication that lists osteoporosis as a possible side effect, steps to prevent bone loss should be taken as soon as your disease is diagnosed or your medication is prescribed.

Type I, or postmenopausal, is the most common type and stems from the loss of estrogen. It typically manifests in fractures within fifteen to twenty years after a woman goes through menopause.

Type II, or senile osteoporosis, is strictly age related and can affect both men and women, usually in their seventh or eighth decade of life.

Type III, the newest classification, is drug-induced osteoporosis. It is caused by certain classes of medications, such as corticosteroids, which are prescribed for unrelated disorders. Type III osteoporosis affects both sexes.

The good news is that for osteoporosis Types I, II, and III, proper treatment and certain lifestyle changes can slow, stop, or even reverse bone loss.

Treating Type IV osteoporosis is more difficult. Type IV is caused by an underlying disease, such as rheumatoid arthritis or inflammatory bowel disease, which may not be curable. In Type IV osteoporosis bone loss is independent of any drugs the patient may be taking to treat the primary condition.

There are two other forms of osteoporosis—juvenile osteoporosis and osteoporosis in young adults—but these conditions are extremely rare.

Osteoporosis and disability

One of the most common fears among older people is that of losing their independence. Nobody wants to be a burden on her loved ones or lose her privacy or freedom. The truth is, people with osteoporosis have a much greater risk of losing their independence than those who have strong skeletons. In fact, only one-half to one-third of hip-fracture patients can expect to regain the self-sufficiency they enjoyed prior to the injury. Fifteen to twenty-five percent of hip-fracture sufferers enter a nursing home shortly after the fracture, and hip-fracture patients comprise about 8 percent of all nursing-home residents. Hip fractures are frequently the result of a fall, and falls are the leading cause of death for people age 65 and older.

"In the best of hands, 40 percent of patients sustaining a hip fracture will not survive two years following that injury," write experts from The Hospital for Special Surgery, Division of Orthopaedic Surgery, at Memorial Sloan-Kettering Cancer Center in New York in the medical textbook *Osteoporosis: Etiology, Diagnosis, and Management* (Raven Press, 1988). "Of the (hip-fracture) patients originating from a nursing home, 70 percent will not survive one year."

In addition to being physically limiting, osteoporotic fractures can be quite painful and disfiguring, especially when fractures involve the vertebrae. Not surprisingly, depression and loss of self-esteem are common occurrences in the osteoporosis population. The emotional aspects of osteoporosis will be discussed in Chapter 9.

OSTEOPOROSIS COMES OF AGE

Until 1984, osteoporosis was virtually unknown by the nonmedical public. That year the National Institutes of Health conducted a Consensus Development Conference, during which the scope of osteoporosis was recognized, and the National Osteoporosis Foundation (NOF) was formed; there has since been a flurry of news reports and several books published on the topic.

In July 1993, Massachusetts established the nation's first statewide osteoporosis education program, according to the fall 1993 NOF newsletter, *The Osteoporosis Report*. The newsletter states that Massachusetts allocated $500,000 to promote greater public awareness about osteoporosis, educate patients and health-care workers about the disease, and identify health professionals who specialize in osteoporosis services. New York, California, Missouri, Illinois, and Maryland have similar bills pending, according to the newsletter, which further notes that, in spring 1993, osteoporosis was identified as "one of the leading diseases of women" by Bernadine Healy, M.D., then director of the National Institutes of Health. Sandra C. Raymond, executive director of the NOF, writes in the newsletter that most people are unable to find medical services "that can help them take the necessary steps to prevent osteoporosis, detect it once it has occurred, or treat it when bone loss threatens to cause or has already caused fractures."

Because of the apparent difficulty people have finding medical advice regarding osteoporosis, the public is vulnerable to certain misunderstandings about the condition. This book aims to clarify those misunderstandings and to put you and your loved ones on the road to better bone health.

MYTHS AND FACTS

MYTH: It's impossible to predict who will develop osteoporosis.

FACT: Doctors have identified a number of risk factors that can give you a fairly good idea of whether you will get osteoporosis. We discuss these risk factors in Chapter 3. In addition, there are a variety of techniques to measure bone density. Abnormally low bone density, the hallmark of osteoporosis, can lead to fractures. Recently, a particular gene type that contains instructions for the vitamin D receptor has been found to be more prevalent in women with osteoporosis. Knowing whether you're at risk gives you an opportunity to take steps to prevent osteoporosis or to lessen its severity.

MYTH: Since osteoporosis is a problem of the elderly, young women need not worry about it.

FACT: Young women and adolescents are in the best position to lower their osteoporosis risk. By getting adequate calcium, vitamin D, and exercise and avoiding tobacco, caffeine, and alcohol, they can build a strong, dense skeleton that can better withstand bone loss in their later years.

MYTH: Once I have osteoporosis, it's too late to do anything about it.

FACT: Even if you've already endured an osteoporotic fracture, there are certain things you can do that might strengthen your skeleton and lower your risk for future fractures. Hormone replacement therapy (HRT) can safely begin years after menopause, for example, and there are exercises you can do that are designed for people with fragile bones. We discuss HRT in Chapter 6 and exercise in Chapter 8.

MYTH: Only women get osteoporosis.

FACT: Osteoporosis is a growing problem for men, too. The NOF says that one in five men will get osteoporosis. Men account for about 15 percent of vertebral fractures and about 20 percent of all hip fractures, according to Bernard A. Roos, M.D., of the Miami Veterans Administration Medical Center. Since men don't undergo menopause, there is no period of dramatic bone loss as there is in women. Men, particularly white and Asian men, do experience a slow, steady decline in spine mineral density after age 40—about 1 percent a year. Between ages 20 and 85, men lose about 25 percent of their overall bone mass. Overt signs of osteoporosis in men don't usually occur until after age 65. As in women, osteoporosis is believed to be linked to the withdrawal of sex hormones. Men are also vulnerable to the same nonhormonal bone-robbing factors as women, such as the use of certain drugs and certain chronic diseases like diabetes and alcoholism.

MYTH: I can prevent osteoporosis simply by taking calcium supplements.

FACT: Any nutritionist will tell you that it is always better to get calcium, or any nutrient, from foods rather than supplements. If you find it difficult to get enough calcium from your diet, your doctor may recommend supplementation. Be aware that calcium intake is only one of several factors in the osteoporosis-prevention equation. Calcium alone may not be adequate to maintain bone mass in the postmenopausal woman. Nutrition is the focus of Chapter 7.

MYTH: Since my bones fracture easily, I should avoid exercising.

FACT: Certain kinds of exercise, such as sit-ups, that strain the back and shoulders should be avoided by osteoporosis sufferers. However, a carefully prescribed routine of low impact aerobic and isometric exercises can reduce your risk of fracture by strengthening your bones and muscles. Physical activity may also help to alleviate pain and improve your sense of balance, which lowers your risk of falling. Chapter 8 is devoted to the topic of exercise.

CHAPTER 2

THE SKELETON: A SURPRISINGLY DYNAMIC ORGAN

The skeleton is commonly associated with lifelessness: a skull and crossbones represents death; the legendary rock group, the Grateful Dead, uses a skeleton as its mascot. But those images belie reality. Your skeleton is not only alive, it is a surprisingly dynamic organ.

The skeleton is a factory for blood cells even as it gives your body form and support. At the same time, your skeleton is busily dissolving old bone tissue and replacing it with new. This constant renewal process, known as remodeling, occurs at the cellular level and is key to understanding osteoporosis. Remodeling is discussed in greater depth later in this chapter.

Remodeling, or reshaping, has been called a "preventive maintenance system" designed to keep bones dense and strong. In osteoporosis, physiologic changes that occur naturally and as a result of outside influences throw the remodeling system so far off balance that bone becomes too thin and prone to fractures under the slightest trauma or simply under the weight of gravity.

Remodeling takes place from infancy on as bone attempts to achieve just the right physical characteristics to support us. Bone increases in length until the end of the adolescent growth spurt, usually the young adult years. Bone continues to increase in thickness until the late twenties to mid-thirties. After about age 35, there is no further increase in bone thickness. The maximum thickness reached at that time is called "peak bone mass." Many researchers believe that we are all born with a genetically determined "potential level" of peak bone mass. Whether your skeleton achieves its full potential is a major influence on your risk of developing osteoporosis later in life.

Several factors seem to determine whether you will reach your maximum potential. The first is probably how much calcium you take in during your growing years. Calcium and other nutritional factors in osteoporosis will be discussed in Chapter 7. How much weight-bearing exercise you get is another factor, which will be explored in Chapter 8. Another determinant of peak bone mass may be the remodeling system itself.

What bone is made of

There are two kinds of bone. About 80 percent of bone is compact or "cortical" bone, which forms the outer shell. Inside the shell is a spongelike bone structure called "trabecular" or "cancellous" bone. Dispersed in trabecular bone is marrow, the soft, fatty tissue where all the red blood cells and platelets and most of the white blood cells are manufactured. Both cortical and trabecular bone can be affected by osteoporosis. But trabecular bone is more vulnerable because of its larger surface area and because remodeling is far more active in trabecular bone compared with the outer shell.

Both cortical and trabecular bone are made primarily of bone collagen. Collagen is a type of protein that is a component of connective tissue. In bone, collagen is laid down by specialized cells to form a matrix. This matrix attracts calcium, a mineral, which is absorbed through the gut from foods or calcium supplements. Once in the bone, calcium combines with phosphorus, oxygen, hydrogen, and other elements to form crystals. These crystals give bone its density and hardness. It's interesting to note that along with calcium, the skeleton also stores such toxic elements as lead, mercury, and even radioactive wastes.

But the amount of toxic elements is minuscule when compared to the amount of calcium in bone.

Ninety-nine percent of the body's calcium can be found in the skeleton. The other one percent is found in the blood and in other bodily fluids that surround cells, the so-called extracellular fluid. One percent may not sound like much. But that tiny amount is essential for life and normal cellular function. Whenever the blood calcium level falls below normal, a hormonal response is initiated, ordering the skeleton to release more calcium into the bloodstream until the extracellular calcium level rises back to normal.

While the amount of calcium you ingest appears to affect the amount of calcium in your skeleton, it has no impact on the amount of calcium in your extracellular fluid, explains Dr. Robert P. Heaney in his book *Calcium and Common Sense* (Doubleday, 1988). Whenever your blood calcium level dips, your body must cannibalize your skeleton to keep you alive. This is one reason calcium is taken from bone.

The skeleton also loses calcium when the remodeling process is thrown off balance. Normally about 25 to 30 percent of trabecular bone is replaced through remodeling per year compared with just 2 to 3 percent of cortical bone. In their book *Osteoporosis: Etiology, Diagnosis, and Management,* experts from Memorial Sloan-Kettering in New York note that "patients with Type I osteoporosis have a rate of trabecular bone loss that is three times greater than that in normal peers."

How bone is remodeled

It is believed that a new remodeling site is activated somewhere in the adult skeleton every ten seconds, according to the textbook. Thousands of these microscopic sites, called "remodeling units," are dispersed throughout the skeleton like islands.

1. Resting Phase

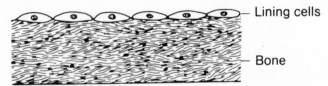

A bone surface is covered by a protective layer of bone cells—called lining cells.

2. Resorption

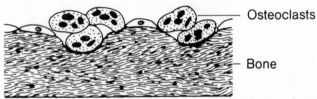

During resorption, osteoclasts (large cells with many nuclei) invade the bone surface and erode it, dissolving the mineral and the matrix.

3. Resorption Complete

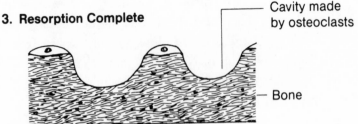

A small cavity is created in the bone surface—resorption complete.

FIGURE 1   Remodeling. From *Osteoporosis: The Silent Thief,* Peck, W., Avioli, L., © 1988. Reprinted with permission from Scott, Foresman and Co. and AARP.

4. Formation—Repair

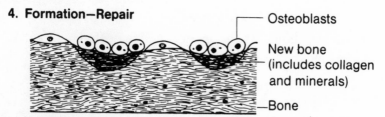

Bone-forming cells begin to fill in the cavity with new bone.

5. Repair Complete

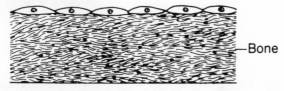

Finally, the bone surface is completely restored.

No one knows what activates the formation of a remodeling unit or why one area of the skeleton is targeted and not another at any given time.

Once a site is activated, specialized cells called "osteoclasts" go to work. Osteoclasts—large cells with many nuclei—form the excavation team, scooping out a portion of bone through a process known as "resorption." In resorption, osteoclasts secrete an acidic chemical that digests, or resorbs, a predetermined amount of bone tissue. In cortical bone, osteoclasts construct a tunnel. In trabecular bone, osteoclasts leave behind a groove.

It takes an estimated two to four weeks for the osteoclasts to complete their work. When the tunnel or groove is completed, other specialized bone cells called "osteoblasts" take over and lay down new bone collagen to replace the tissue that was resorbed. The collagen attracts calcium and other minerals to form crystals. Within a few months, the tunnel or groove is filled in with new bone. At that point, the remodeling unit enters a "resting phase."

Bone cell tug-of-war

In a sense, osteoclasts and osteoblasts are in a constant tug-of-war. From childhood through adolescence, the osteoblasts usually win, so the buildup of new bone outpaces the resorption of old. Many factors can influence the activity of osteoclasts and osteoblasts, including hormonal ones. For example, it appears that estrogen is largely responsible for achieving bone growth by stimulating bone-building cells to send a turn-off signal to bone-resorbing cells. This role played by estrogen may partially explain why girls experience a growth spurt around the time of puberty. It also explains why older women experience a spell of accelerated bone loss after menopause.

Also influencing osteoblasts and osteoclasts are local growth factors (substances produced in the area where bone is being formed); physical factors, such as how much weight-bearing physical activity an individual gets; and nutritional factors. Weight-bearing exercise, such as walking, is any physical activity whereby bone and muscle must work against gravitational forces on a repetitive basis.

In adulthood, up to age 30 to 35, the tug-of-war becomes a draw as the remodeling process enters a phase of equilibrium: the same amount of bone is taken away as is built up. This equilibrium process between the osteoclasts and the osteoblasts is known as "coupling."

After age 40, osteoclasts and osteoblasts begin "uncoupling" as the osteoclasts start winning the tug-of-war. The result: The skeleton begins to lose more bone than it creates. The cumulative effect of what is happening in each bone unit determines whether the person will develop osteoporosis.

It may help to think of your skeleton as a bank account. During childhood through young adulthood, you are building up your savings account by making as many deposits and as few withdrawals as possible. From your early twenties to age 35 to 40, you are putting in as much money as you are taking out. But as you approach menopause, your withdrawals begin to outstrip your deposits. After menopause, your withdrawals get bigger and your deposits get even smaller. If you had enough money in the bank to begin with, you won't overdraft your account. If your savings were below what they should have been, however, you'll begin bouncing checks. And that sets you up for trouble ahead.

How much bone is lost varies among individuals. In general, those with the densest peak bone mass withstand the loss better than those who never reached their full skeletal potential. In men, bone loss generally continues at a slow pace until their seventies or eighties. In women, bone loss accelerates markedly for several years after their periods stop. Research has shown that most women lose 2 to 3 percent of bone per year for five to eight years immediately following menopause. That amounts to 10 percent to almost 25 percent of bone being lost in a relatively short time span, due to estrogen depletion. Add bone loss solely due to aging factors, and over the years bone density can diminish up to 20 to 30 percent in men and 40 to 50 percent in women.

There are a number of theories as to why an imbalance between osteoclast and osteoblast activity occurs as people age. David W. Dempster, Ph.D., of Columbia University's Helen Hayes Hospital, notes that "the slow, age-related bone loss is thought to be primarily due to osteoblastic insufficiency.

"With each successive remodeling cycle, the osteoblasts become less and less efficient at refilling the resorption cavities,"

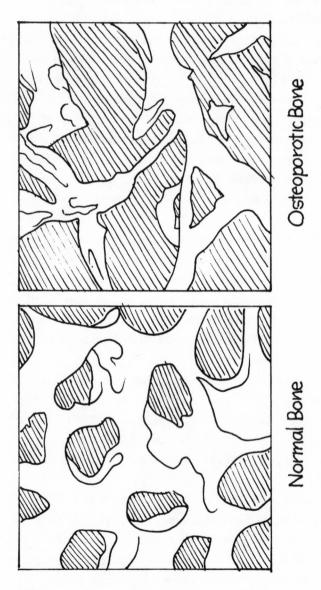

FIGURE 2   Normal bone vs. osteoporotic bone. The drawing on the left shows the internal structure of healthy bone. Note the thick bridges of trabeculae (hardened collagen and protein) between the pores. On the right, note the bone weakened by osteoporosis. The pores are much larger and the trabeculae are thin and fragile.

he reported to a 1993 medical conference on osteoporosis. Partially filled cavities would lead to a gradual thinning of trabecular bone. Another possibility noted in the medical textbook *Disorders of Bone and Mineral Metabolism* (Raven Press, 1992) is that in older skeletons there is a delay between the time resorption is completed and formation begins.

Rapid postmenopausal bone loss is thought to stem from overworking osteoclasts, according to Dr. Dempster. "Following menopause, the osteoclasts become hyperactive, penetrate too far into the trabecular plates and perforate them. . . . Clearly, this is a much more detrimental form of bone loss in terms of structural integrity and mechanical strength."

Learning to manipulate bone remodeling cycles holds great promise for the future of osteoporosis therapy and is the basis of some experimental therapies. Some current osteoporosis treatments aim either to stimulate osteoblasts to make bone or to inhibit osteoclasts from resorbing bone.

CHAPTER 3

ARE YOU AT RISK FOR OSTEOPOROSIS?

If you're seriously trying to reduce your risk for heart disease, you won't just cut some fat out of your diet. You'll also step up your exercise program, avoid red meat, take a stress-reduction class, lose weight, give up cigarettes, and maybe even take drugs to lower your cholesterol level or reduce high blood pressure. You'd take a multifaceted prevention strategy because heart disease has been linked to a variety of risk factors.

The same holds true for osteoporosis. A variety of risk factors, the most important one being the loss of estrogen, has been implicated in osteoporosis. Some risk factors, such as ancestry and genes, are beyond your control. Others, such as failing to get enough calcium from your diet, are very much under your control. As an added bonus, many steps you take to lower your risk for osteoporosis—such as quitting smoking and getting enough exercise—also help to protect your heart and improve your overall health. This chapter will cover the many factors that can either increase your chances of developing osteoporosis or protect you from it. For those who have already been diagnosed with osteoporosis and suffered one or more fractures, this chapter will provide tips on lowering your risk of breaking a bone in the future.

RISK FACTORS FOR OSTEOPOROSIS

Sex and age

Women have a higher risk of osteoporosis simply by virtue of their sex. In Western societies at least, women generally have smaller bones than men and therefore don't have as much calcium in their skeletons. Women also undergo menopause. During menopause, women experience a relatively abrupt and dramatic falloff of the female sex hormone estrogen. Among other things, estrogen helps to preserve bone density.

In men, it is the male sex hormone, testosterone, that helps maintain bone density. The amount of testosterone produced by the male body withdraws very gradually in old age. As a result, medical records show that the number of hip fractures among elderly women, for example, is two to three times higher than among elderly men. Fractures of the wrist and other bones are six to eight times higher in women.

Hormones play one role in bone density. Age plays another. Both men and women experience a slow decrease in bone density with age that appears to be independent of hormone levels. Researchers can't fully explain it. Like wrinkles and gray hair, loss of bone density seems to be a normal consequence of aging.

Heredity

Generally speaking, thin women with small frames and fair complexions face a higher risk of osteoporosis than women with larger frames or dark complexions. This is probably because skeletal frame and body weight are usually inherited. If your mother or grandmother was diagnosed with osteoporosis (or lost two or more inches of height after age 60), you should probably consider yourself at risk for osteoporosis.

Recently, scientists identified a more tangible hereditary

link. A study, which appeared in the scientific journal *Nature* in January 1994, was the first to point to an identifiable genetic link between a specific gene and osteoporosis. While the findings are still preliminary, there is hope that one day a test may be performed to discover early on whether a woman is genetically predisposed to osteoporosis.

Race

No one knows exactly why, but African-Americans have more bone mass and greater bone density throughout their skeletons than whites, and black women suffer fewer fractures than white women do. In fact, black women are only half as likely to suffer a hip fracture as Caucasian and Asian women. To figure out why, a 1991 study, reported in the *New England Journal of Medicine,* measured spinal bone density of black and white girls and found little difference until puberty. At puberty, black girls had a 34 percent increase in bone density compared with just 11 percent in white girls. Another study found that bone density at various skeletal sites was greater in black children than in white children ages 7 through 12. Commenting in *Current Opinion in Rheumatology 1993,* French researchers Patricia Dargent, Ph.D., and Gerard Breart, M.D., suggest that differences in spinal bone density between black and white women may stem from hormonal and metabolic differences during adolescence. As our understanding of the relationship between genes and osteoporosis increases, doctors may better understand the racial difference in risk for osteoporosis.

Estrogen loss

When estrogen levels decline, bone loss accelerates. This phenomenon is well documented in postmenopausal women and in women who have had their ovaries surgically removed. Women lose about 3 percent of their bone mass annually during the five to ten years that follow menopause, compared with about 1 percent a year for premenopausal women after age 35. Taking estrogen replacement therapy can help avoid postmenopausal bone loss. But, as you will see in Chapter 6, estrogen therapy carries its own risks.

Inadequate calcium intake

Bone health is largely dependent on getting adequate daily calcium throughout life, particularly in the early teens. Research suggests that women who were calcium deficient in their youth may never achieve their full bone mass potential. Women who are lactose intolerant (lacking the enzymes necessary to digest milk sugars) tend to be the most calcium deficient because they cannot eat dairy products, which are the richest sources of dietary calcium. Insufficient bone density can set these women up for osteoporotic fractures in the future. The daily requirement for calcium changes with age, pregnancy, and lactation status. Yet very few women ingest enough calcium any time during their lives to build and maintain strong skeletons. In fact, in June 1994, a panel of experts assembled by the National Institutes of Health reported that fifty percent of American women and men are calcium deficient by the time they reach adulthood.

Other dietary factors

Diets that are high in insoluble fiber or include excessive amounts of protein can impede the intestine's ability to absorb calcium. Both fiber and protein molecules bind with calcium and carry the mineral out of the body before it can be used. If you are on a high-fiber diet, which is believed to reduce the risk for colon cancer and other diseases, make sure your intake of calcium-rich foods is equally high.

Anorexia and bulimia

Anorexia nervosa is a disease marked by self-starvation. People with bulimia go through cycles of binging then purging what they ate by forcing themselves to vomit or by abusing laxatives. Most anorexia and bulimia sufferers are teenage girls and young women. Anorexics and bulimics deprive their bodies of vital bone-building nutrients at the very time that they should be getting adequate nutrition. In addition to the nutrition-related bone loss, anorexics often get insufficient bone-protecting estrogen because they lose so much body fat. The body needs a certain amount of fat in order to produce an adequate level of estrogen. Even more disturbing, anorexics may be unable to make up for the bone loss, even if they take calcium supplements during the period of their eating disorder or after their recovery, according to a study out of the Children's National Medical Center in Washington. The study by Tomas Silber, M.D., published in the *Journal of Pediatrics* in September 1993, looked at seven teenage girls with anorexia and found that they were unable to absorb calcium into their bone even when they were getting enough calcium through their diets. Dr. Silber surmised that the problem stemmed from low levels of estrogen or elevated levels of cortisol, a body chemical used in stress management.

Lack of vitamin D

Even if you religiously ingest 1,500 milligrams (mg) of calcium a day, much of it will pass right through you if you are deficient in vitamin D. Milk is fortified with vitamin D. Another way to build up your stores of vitamin D is through exposing your skin to small doses of sunshine. Radiation from the sun helps the body to make vitamin D, which enables the intestine to absorb bone-building calcium from foods. In fact, studies have shown that accelerated bone loss can occur during the winter months, particularly in northern latitudes. Seasonal bone loss is reversible, however. Elderly women who are inclined to spend all their time indoors should be encouraged to get some sun as often as possible, at least fifteen minutes a day. Sunscreens should be utilized during more prolonged sun exposure.

Sedentary lifestyle

Women who get little or no exercise appear to be at higher risk for osteoporosis than women who engage in weight-bearing exercise, such as low-impact aerobics, volleyball, or racquet sports, on a *regular* basis. (A more strenuous exercise, such as running or jogging, should be undertaken only by those fit enough to participate without injury; consult your doctor.) This fact cannot be overemphasized: Exercise can help in the battle against osteoporosis only when it is properly and persistently performed. Further, women should keep in mind that while the health benefits of swimming are many, it is not weight-bearing and probably does not help prevent osteoporosis unless it is performed extremely vigorously; studies are being done on this issue.

People who are bedridden can lose up to 1 percent of their trabecular bone per week. Astronauts can lose that much bone while weightless in space. As soon as the bedridden person resumes normal physical activity and the astronaut is back on Earth, bone loss is reversed. On the flip side, athletic people, such as tennis players and professional dancers, tend to have denser, thicker bone in the limbs they use most. Too much vigorous exercise among women, however, has been associated with reduced spinal bone density, probably because these athletes stop menstruating, because their estrogen levels have fallen too low.

Alcohol

As if alcoholics didn't have enough problems, their frequent imbibing may also poison their bones, animal and human research suggests. The toxic effect of alcohol seems to reduce the rate of bone formation and mineralization, notes Daniel Schapira, M.D., a rheumatology consultant at Rambam Medical Center in Haifa, Israel. Alcoholics also tend to have calcium-deficient diets, he points out in a review article that appears in *Seminars in Arthritis and Rheumatism* (June 1990). Alcoholism may impair the body's ability to absorb the calcium it does get partly because chronic drinking reduces the amount of parathyroid hormone and vitamin D in the bloodstream. Dr. Schapira's article also points to increased loss of minerals, such as calcium, in the urine of heavy drinkers. Making matters worse, alcoholics have a tendency to be heavy smokers and may be unable to engage in regular exercise, two more osteoporosis risk factors. Drunkenness also affects balance, making alcoholics more prone to falling. Not surprisingly, there is an increased fracture rate among alcoholics, which Dr. Schapira calls an "important health problem and a significant burden to society."

"Osteoporosis should be suspected in every chronic alcohol abuser, regardless of the other medical consequences of alcoholism," Dr. Schapira advises physicians, adding that even "sporadic alcohol ingestion should arouse suspicion."

Smoking

In addition to increasing a person's risk for heart disease, a variety of cancers, and other health problems, smoking may also contribute to osteoporosis. Cigarettes have been linked to diminished bone mass in premenopausal women and accelerated bone loss in postmenopausal women. Possible reasons: Tobacco is thought to affect estrogen metabolism and curtail calcium absorption, according to researchers at the Calcium and Bone Metabolism Laboratory at Tufts University. "Smoking also has been associated with earlier menopause and low body weight, both of which are independent risk factors for osteoporosis," the researchers write in a 1993 article in *Osteoporosis International*.

Caffeine

It's not proven, but there is some circumstantial evidence that a diet excessive in caffeine may be a contributing factor in the development of osteoporosis. The most well-known sources of caffeine are coffee and tea. There are also hidden sources, such as chocolate and certain colas and other sodas. If you have osteoporosis or are at risk of developing it, and you must have your morning caffeine fix, try to limit consumption to one or two cups a day or skip a day here and there. You can also wean yourself off coffee by drinking a fifty-fifty mixture of caffeinated and decaf. There are no set guidelines on how much caffeine you can have without raising your osteoporosis risk, but it's probably sustained exposure to caffeine rather than episodic exposure that's the culprit.

Older women who are longtime coffee drinkers may be able to offset bone loss by drinking milk regularly, a 1994 study by the University of California, San Diego, found. The study, published in the *Journal of the American Medical Association*, asked 980 women ages 50 to 98 about their lifetime dietary habits. Measurements of hip and spine density showed that coffee drinkers who drank one or more glasses of milk daily had 6.5 percent more bone density compared to those who drank two cups of coffee daily but no milk.

Medications

Certain medications are known to quicken bone loss or otherwise cause bone to lose density. One is long-term steroid therapy, prescribed for such ailments as rheumatoid arthritis, asthma, inflammatory bowel disease, and lupus. Corticosteroids, such as prednisone, can cause both trabecular and cortical bone loss by repressing the generation of new osteoblasts and inhibiting their ability to build bone. Steroids also increase the amount of calcium excreted in urine and reduce the intestine's ability to absorb calcium from food. Corticosteroids accelerate trabecular bone loss, which makes patients more prone to fractures of the vertebrae, ribs, and possibly the hips. Urinalyses of patients on corticosteroids show that the drug rapidly snatches calcium out of bone soon after therapy begins, but later this effect stabilizes. Nonetheless, users continue to have a negative calcium balance and to lose bone mass until they stop taking the drug. Some corticosteroid users are more susceptible than others to bone loss.

Other drugs that appear to diminish bone mass include anticoagulants, including heparin (long-term use); certain diuretics; chronic lithium therapy; chemotherapy; anticonvulsant drugs; tetracycline; and cyclosporine A, which is taken by some organ-transplant patients to prevent rejection.

People with low calcium intake who use aluminum-containing antacids may face an elevated risk of osteoporosis. In many cases, bone density returns to normal after the drugs are withdrawn.

Excessive doses of thyroid hormone may diminish cortical bone mass, although usual doses may offer some protection against fractures. Thyroid hormone is widely prescribed in this country, albeit sometimes unnecessarily. It used to be given to women as a placebo to help with everything from fatigue to depression. That practice is less common today. But even when thyroid hormone is taken for legitimate purposes—to compensate for an underactive thyroid gland, for instance—many women still take too much. A dose of thyroid hormone that is only mildly excessive can rob calcium from bone if taken over the course of many years.

Jane, who has osteoporosis and an underactive thyroid gland, deliberately takes a higher dose of thyroid hormone than was prescribed to treat her thyroid deficiency. Why? To keep her weight down, she says, even though she isn't fat. Despite a long discussion with her doctor about the dangers of osteoporosis, Jane refuses to reduce her thyroid dosage. Letting vanity get the best of her, she appears willing to risk fractures in order to keep her weight down five to ten pounds. Weight gain can be seen in a mirror. Bone loss is invisible but potentially far more danger-ous than a few extra pounds.

Cushing's syndrome

Most common in middle age, Cushing's syndrome occurs when overactive adrenal glands pump too much cortisonelike chemicals into the bloodstream. The syndrome can be caused by prolonged use of corticosteroid drugs, enlargement of the adre-nal glands, or a tumor in the pituitary gland (the pituitary con-trols adrenal function). In addition to weakened bones, the syndrome can cause obesity, wasted limbs, acne, stretch marks, easy bruising, increased body hair, mental depression, paranoia, or even euphoria.

If drug-induced, Cushing's syndrome can be alleviated by slowly withdrawing the corticosteroids. If there is a tumor in the adrenals or if the adrenals are enlarged, the glands can be removed. Pituitary tumors can either be removed surgically or shrunk by radiation and drug treatment.

Turner's syndrome

Turner's syndrome is a chromosomal abnormality in which girls fail to produce estrogen and therefore never mature through puberty. The disorder affects about 1 in 3,000 girls and can be treated with estrogen therapy.

Other medical disorders

Osteoporosis has been associated with chronic obstructive lung diseases, including emphysema and bronchitis; acromegaly, a rare disease marked by the enlargement of the jaw, skull, hands, and feet; Graves' disease (thyrotoxicosis), a toxic condition stemming from an overactive thyroid gland; insulin-dependent diabetes; mastocytosis, a rare skin disease marked by itchy, yellowish swellings usually found on the trunk; rheumatoid arthritis; and endometriosis, a condition in which tissue that normally grows inside the uterus each month also appears outside it.

FACTORS THAT RAISE YOUR RISK OF FRACTURE

While a plethora of factors can lay the groundwork for osteoporosis, fragile bones won't hurt you if they remain intact. Lowering your risk of falling, then, becomes the most important issue if your bone density has fallen below normal or you've already been diagnosed with osteoporosis.

Here are some steps you can take to lower your risk of falling:

Make your environment safe

Make sure all throw rugs have rubber backings. Tape down or hide loose electrical cords. Use nonskid tape in the tub instead of a bath mat. Install grab bars in your bathrooms. Be sure your vacuum cleaner's handle is long enough so that you can stand upright while vacuuming. Repair unstable furniture. Be sure stairwells are well lit. Use night lights. Wear shoes with rubberized soles, especially when walking on smooth floors. Fix uneven sidewalks near your home. Be extra cautious going in and out of buses and when walking in supermarkets and other stores where floors can be especially slippery. Don't stand on chairs to grab things. Keep things on lower shelves or ask for help if you can't reach something.

Beware of drugs that impair balance

Many medications cause dizziness or fatigue, which can increase your risk of falling. Among these are antihistamines, sleeping pills, muscle relaxers, and certain hypertension medications.

Hypnotic (psychotropic) drugs that remain active in the body for more than twenty-four hours appear to be the most dangerous, according to an investigation by Wayne A. Ray, Ph.D., and his colleagues at Vanderbilt University School of Medicine. The most common ones are long-acting tranquilizers, such as flurazepam (Dalmane and Durapam), diazepam (Valium), and chlordiazepoxide (Librium). Other drugs associated with increased falling and fracture risks are tricyclic antidepressants and antipsychotics, according to Dr. Ray. The study, which involved more than 5,700 elderly people, found that the higher the dose, the higher the fracture risk. These findings appeared in the February 12, 1987, issue of the *New England Journal of Medicine*.

Superwoman syndrome

Skiers know that they are more prone to falling on the slopes toward the end of the day than in the beginning. The main reason is fatigue. Fatigue is also a culprit in many falls among osteoporotic women. If you have osteoporosis yet continue to do all the housework, shopping, and playing with the grandchildren, you may be setting yourself up for a fall. Cutting back on your obligations and resting or napping at least once a day can keep your energy level up and your fall risk down.

Alcohol

Aside from the potential bone-robbing effects of alcohol, drinking can impair your balance. Also, small amounts of alcohol can interact with certain medications to cause dizziness and other problems.

Ear infections

Disorders of the inner or middle ear can cause dizziness or vertigo and impair balance. These disorders include labyrinthitis, an inflammation of the inner ear; Ménière's disease, marked by abnormally high pressure in the fluid of the inner ear; and otitis media, an inflammation of the middle ear, according to the American Medical Association's *Encyclopedia of Medicine*.

Effects of aging

As people age, their reaction time, sense of balance, and coordination naturally decline. Decreased muscle tone, decreased strength, and declining flexibility among the elderly can impede their ability to catch themselves before falling.

Getting up too quickly

To avoid dizziness, try not to get up too quickly after you finish eating, sleeping, or resting.

Failing eyesight

Declining vision is another common consequence of aging. If your eyesight is diminished, it's even more important to keep your home free of hazards. Get your eyes examined annually.

Stroke

A stroke, or a tumor, that affects the part of the brain known as the cerebellum may cause clumsiness of the arms and legs.

Other disorders

A number of other diseases can raise your risk of falling by producing a clumsy gait. They include spinal-cord damage stemming from syphilis, tumors of the spine, nerve damage due to a vitamin B_{12} deficiency, and certain vascular disorders, according to the *Encyclopedia of Medicine*.

FACTORS THAT MAY PROTECT YOU AGAINST OSTEOPOROSIS

Hormone replacement therapy (HRT), proper calcium nutrition, and weight-bearing exercise are the primary features of an osteoporosis-prevention program. These topics will be explored in detail later in this book. Here are other factors that may offer some protection against osteoporosis.

Adequate body weight

Although the risks for heart disease and other illnesses rise in obese people, it is believed that being 10 percent or more over your ideal weight offers some measure of protection against osteoporosis. For one thing, obese people exert more energy to undertake daily activities. Also, fat cells can make bone-preserving estrogen even after menopause. Health experts don't advocate being obese, of course, but if you are underweight, it's a good idea to gain enough pounds so that your weight is normal for your height and build.

Muscularity

Muscle tissue can serve as a buffer for bones during falls. What's more, people with strong muscles have a greater ability to catch themselves before they hit the floor. Muscle tissue also may produce some estrogen. Chapter 8 will describe a variety of exercises designed to strengthen your muscles and skeleton.

Pregnancy

In pregnancy, a woman's ability to absorb calcium from food increases to ensure that both she and her fetus get enough of this vital mineral.

Late menopause

The majority of women go through menopause between the ages of 45 and 55. Women who stop menstruating in their mid-fifties or later have a lower risk for osteoporosis since they produce estrogen for a longer period of time.

Hip pads

Wearing hip pads has been shown to offer a measure of protection against hip fractures among frail, elderly osteoporosis patients.

CHAPTER 4

FINDING A DOCTOR

When you have arthritis, you go to a rheumatologist. When you have cancer, you go to an oncologist. When you need a Pap test, you visit your gynecologist. And when you have a plantar wart, a podiatrist stands ready to treat you.

But when you have osteoporosis, to whom do you turn? Despite the fact that osteoporosis is one of the largest and most costly public health problems in the United States today, there is no single medical discipline that specializes in osteoporosis.

The good news is that since the mid-1980s all physicians who treat women and senior citizens have been urged by their respective professional societies to educate their patients about osteoporosis. The public, meanwhile, is becoming increasingly aware of osteoporosis primarily due to media interest in the disorder. Many newspapers, magazines, and television news shows have begun to cover major findings in osteoporosis research because so many of their readers and viewers are affected. One poll showed that public awareness of the existence of osteoporosis has increased from 15 to 85 percent in recent years.

Articles about osteoporosis have appeared in a spectrum of medical journals, including *Fertility and Sterility, Metabolism, Annals of Internal Medicine, Clinical Endocrinology, New England Journal of Medicine, Journal of Nutrition, Annals of the New York Academy of Sciences, Southern Medical Journal, Journal of the American Paraplegia Society, Annals of Rhematological Diseases, Arthritis and Rheumatism, Journal of*

Adolescent Health, Bone, American Journal of Nursing, Journal of Sports Medicine and Physical Fitness, Metabolism, Primary Care, and *Orthopaedic Clinics of North America.* There is even a journal solely devoted to osteoporosis, *Osteoporosis International,* which is co-sponsored by the National Osteoporosis Foundation. Clearly, osteoporosis has become the subject of intense scientific investigation in the United States and abroad.

Periodically, medical journals publish review articles. The authors of these articles examine reams of research studies, synthesize the information, and draw conclusions based on the latest available data. By condensing the findings of numerous studies into one summary, these articles provide doctors with handy references to help them prescribe the most effective and safest treatments for their patients.

Physicians seeking more current information can attend any of a number of osteoporosis conferences held throughout the year around the United States and Europe. At these meetings lectures are presented by researchers who have devoted their life's work to understanding bone metabolism and osteoporosis. Conference attendees also have a chance to learn what doctors in other cities and countries are doing to help their osteoporosis patients.

Research findings are sometimes conflicting or inconclusive, which leads to disagreement over the best treatment approaches. As a patient, you must seek out a doctor who keeps up with the ever-broadening scientific knowledge base and state-of-the-art treatment protocols, which are continually being refined as scientists learn more about the nature of bone and osteoporosis. But successful treatment does not lie in your doctor's hands alone. By educating yourself about osteoporosis, you have a better chance of making any treatment approach more successful. Reading this book is an excellent way to increase your knowledge base and become a more savvy consumer of medical services.

Who treats osteoporosis?

Family practitioners, endocrinologists, internists, OB-GYNs, rheumatologists, and orthopedists—virtually all doctors who treat women or senior citizens—are likely to encounter patients with osteoporosis. Osteoporosis may not even be the reason the patient sought medical attention in the first place.

Today all primary-care physicians are urged to look for signs of osteoporosis in their older patients and to educate all of their female patients about osteoporosis prevention. Risk assessment for osteoporosis should be routine as a woman enters menopause. If your doctor hasn't talked with you about osteoporosis, you may want to bring up the topic yourself during your next checkup. If your doctor is unable to give you the information you need or seems uncomfortable discussing osteoporosis, you may opt to find a doctor who is better informed. With all the information available to them, primary-care physicians have scant excuse for failing to "bone up" on what's happening in the world of osteoporosis.

The Washington, D.C.–based National Osteoporosis Foundation may be able to help you locate a physician in your community who treats osteoporosis. An individual membership in the foundation costs $10 a year. As a member, you gain access to a variety of literature. The foundation's address and phone number appear at the end of this book.

Another potential source is your local hospital. Many hospitals offer a physician-referral service that may be able to point you in the right direction. A nearby rehabilitation hospital may also be able to provide you with the names of physicians and allied health professionals experienced in osteoporosis treatment.

The best referral, however, will probably come from a friend, colleague, or relative who has been successfully treated for osteoporosis. If you have osteoporosis or believe you are at risk, let the people in your life know. Word of mouth can work wonders. If you are afraid of being stigmatized, remember that you are not alone. More than 25 million Americans have osteoporosis. Be one of the savvy ones and do something about it.

If possible, get the names of two or three physicians and interview each by phone or in person before seeing him or her as a patient. Are you put on hold and left there for an unusually long time? Does the doctor return your call within a reasonable time frame? Does the doctor explain things in lay terms or in medical jargon? How many osteoporosis patients are presently in the doctor's practice? How successful has he or she been in helping patients stabilize bone density? Has the doctor been able to alleviate the osteoporosis patients' pain, both mental and physical? Can the doctor arrange for you to speak with one of those patients? Does the doctor keep abreast of the latest osteoporosis research findings? Has he or she attended any osteoporosis conferences? What is the doctor's philosophy on hormone replacement therapy as a means of combating osteoporosis? These are some pertinent questions to consider.

You may also wish to ask whether the physician has access to state-of-the-art bone-density measuring equipment. Bone-density measuring equipment is very helpful but not critical in diagnosing osteoporosis; however, it is the only definitive way to diagnose osteopenia, the condition in which bone has lost density but has not yet reached the fracture zone.

Another area of questioning is whether the doctor refers osteoporosis patients to allied health professionals or uses the so-called multidisciplinary, or team, approach to osteoporosis.

WHAT OTHER HEALTH
PROFESSIONALS CAN DO

Francis J. Bonner, Jr., M.D., of the Graduate Hospital in Philadelphia, who works with many osteoporosis patients, is among those who advocate a team approach to rehabilitation for osteoporosis sufferers. The team approach works best when the primary physician and all of the allied health professionals communicate with one another to develop a comprehensive, ongoing program for the patient. These "community intervention" programs have been shown to be successful in preventing falls. Your doctor may refer you to one or more team members or you may request a referral. Here is a modified version of Dr. Bonner's list of potential members of your team and how they can help:

Physiatrist

A physiatrist is a medical doctor who prescribes and coordinates the rehabilitation effort. The physiatrist does this by identifying risk factors for fractures and prescribing exercises, orthotic devices, wheelchairs, canes, walkers, and medications, as needed.

Physical therapist

Under the direction of the primary physician and often in consultation with an occupational therapist, the physical therapist (PT) shows you how to avoid fractures by ensuring that your home and workplace are safe and "ergonomically correct." This phrase means that your furniture, appliances, and other surroundings put little or no stress on your body. The PT also instructs you on an individualized exercise or movement-therapy program to improve your balance and strengthen your muscles in an effort to protect fragile bones.

Occupational therapist

An occupational therapist (OT) retrains you to perform your daily activities with an emphasis on safety awareness. You will also learn from the OT how to conserve energy to avoid fatigue. If needed, the OT will provide adaptive equipment and modifications inside and outside your home.

Rehabilitation nurse/social worker

These professionals evaluate the home for safety, provide medication instruction, coordinate home health services, and act as liaison between medical and allied medical staff.

Nurse practitioner/physician's assistant

As liaisons between the patient and the primary physician, these professionals make sure you understand your condition and help you comply with your treatment. For example, the nurse practitioner or physician's assistant can explain calcium supplements and help you make lifestyle changes geared toward preserving bone or avoiding fractures. The nurse practitioner or physician's assistant reviews side effects of medications you are taking, finds out if you have help at home and whether you have access to exercise equipment or facilities, and brings this information back to the doctor. The nurse practitioner or physician's assistant is usually more readily available when you phone the doctor's office with questions.

Geriatrician

A geriatrician specializes in diseases that commonly strike the elderly. The geriatrician is skilled at developing a treatment and rehabilitation plan appropriate for older people, who may have multiple medical problems. The geriatrician usually has contacts in various social-service agencies and volunteer organizations that are devoted to helping older people remain independent.

Nutritionist

A nutritionist, usually a registered dietitian, can help you choose foods that are high in calcium and vitamin D. The nutritionist can also suggest recipes and meal plans to ensure that you get enough calcium in your diet every day.

Psychotherapist

A psychotherapist aims to help patients regain self-esteem and recover from depression. As you will see in Chapter 9, people with osteoporosis are at high risk for depression and self-esteem problems.

CHAPTER 5

DIAGNOSING OSTEOPOROSIS

Osteoporosis is like a pickpocket who follows his victim from place to place, stealing a penny at a time. Eventually, when she has lost enough money, the victim will realize that she has been robbed. Only if the pickpocket is identified and convicted can his victim hope to regain the money that was stolen. At the very least, she can enroll in a self-defense class or take other steps to protect herself from future robberies.

Like the pickpocket, osteoporosis silently robs its victims of bone, a little at a time. Like the pickpocket's victim, a woman with thinning bones can live normally for decades until she realizes her problem. In the absence of routine bone-density screening programs, almost all osteoporosis patients don't discover that they have a bone problem until their first fracture. Had thinning bones been diagnosed earlier, she could have taken a number of steps to protect herself against bone loss. Once she enters the so-called fracture zone, she can no longer stave off osteoporosis. She can only work toward preventing the next fracture, just as the pickpocket's victim can stash her remaining pennies in a money belt to prevent future thefts.

Taking our analogy one step further, the doctor can be likened to a police officer. In the best of all worlds, the officer will catch the pickpocket red-handed before his robberies make a noticeable dent in his victim's wallet. In the best of all worlds, your doctor will diagnose bone loss early and prescribe treatments and lifestyle changes to keep you from suffering a fracture.

From the doctor's standpoint, diagnosing osteopenia, the precursor to osteoporosis, is the biggest challenge. For one thing, the doctor may not even see the patient until she suffers a fracture. Or the patient will have several vertebral fractures but experience no pain and look normal.

To diagnose bone loss early, gynecologists and other primary-care physicians should suspect possible osteopenia in all female patients over age 40. Your doctor may do a formal osteoporosis risk assessment when you begin menopause, if not sooner. If you are found to be at high risk for osteoporosis, there are a number of tests that can quantify current bone density and help the doctor prescribe preventive treatments.

According to the medical textbook *Osteoporosis: Etiology, Diagnosis, and Management,* all patients who experience an osteoporotic fracture should undergo a "comprehensive medical evaluation." Among other things, this evaluation should reveal whether your osteoporosis is a primary disease, a consequence of an underlying illness, or drug-induced.

The evaluation also assesses the extent of bone loss and fractures and provides baseline measurements that can be used to gauge the effectiveness of subsequent treatment.

Family and personal history

Your doctor will take your history by either having you fill out a questionnaire or asking you a list of questions. In either case, those questions will cover whether your mother or grandmother had osteoporosis or displayed symptoms of the disorder; how many children you had and whether you breast-fed and for how long; at what age you began menstruating and your age at menopause (if relevant); whether menopause was natural or surgical; what, if any, medications, such as corticosteroids, you take and for how long; whether you or any of your blood relatives has a medical problem that is associated with osteoporosis; and your surgical history. Be sure to disclose all surgeries you have had since childhood. Seemingly unrelated surgery can have a powerful impact on your bone density. For example, stomach or intestinal surgery may diminish your ability to absorb calcium.

Your doctor will be particularly interested in any history of cancer because it can influence your treatment dramatically. Women who have had breast cancer, for instance, may be discouraged from taking estrogen after menopause (see Chapter 6). Your doctor also needs to know about any food allergies or sensitivities you may have; whether you smoke; and your levels of alcohol consumption, sun exposure, and physical activity. The doctor will probably ask about your past and present eating habits, paying particular attention to foods that contain bone-building calcium.

Your doctor may even ask you to keep track of how much milk and other calcium-rich foods you ingest over the course of a typical week. This exercise helps the doctor determine whether you are getting enough calcium from your diet and whether supplements are indicated. At the same time, keeping track of your calcium intake can't help but raise your awareness of how important this mineral is to your bone health.

Physical examination

During your physical exam, your doctor will weigh you, measure your height, estimate your fat-to-muscle ratio, and label your skeletal build as small, medium, or large. The doctor may also measure your height while you are sitting, from the top of your head to your buttocks. In compression fractures of the vertebrae, loss of height occurs only in the vertebral column, with hip-to-heel length remaining constant. This measurement can be kept in your medical chart for comparison with future measurements.

The doctor may ask you to stand and walk to examine your posture, leg length, and whether your pelvis is tilted or rotated. You should also mention any muscular pain you may be experiencing. Poor posture or curvature of the spine, pain in certain muscle groups, and disparity in leg length may point to disorders of the spine associated with advanced osteoporosis.

In addition, the doctor will take note of your hair and skin color since fair-skinned, fair-haired individuals are more prone to osteoporosis. Because some people with severe osteoporosis also have thin skin, the doctor may look to see if your skin has a bluish tint. Thin skin can be a sign of corticosteroid drug excess or of osteoporosis associated disorders, such as Cushing's syndrome.

X-rays

X-rays of the upper and lower spine are routine in the diagnostic workup for osteoporosis. X-rays help the doctor detect any deformities or fractures in the vertebrae and identify the cause of muscular back pain. Spinal X-rays also serve as a baseline to compare with future X-rays.

Laboratory tests

If you already have osteoporosis, you will probably have some blood drawn and provide a urine sample as part of your examination. Various tests on blood and urine help measure bone turnover rates and calcium levels. A blood-chemistry profile measures your overall health status as well as your blood-calcium level. Other blood tests measure sex hormone levels, which assess your menopausal status and tell your physician how much bone-protecting hormone your body is producing. A

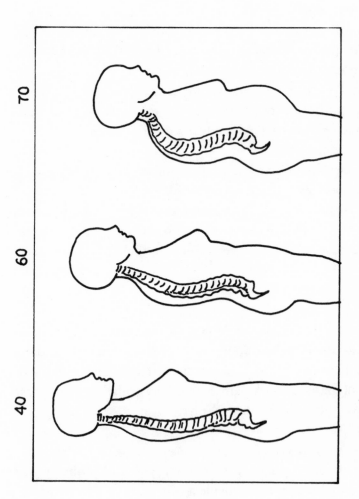

FIGURE 3 Postural changes in women with osteoporosis. The dreaded "dowager's hump" that results from osteoporosis develops gradually, over decades, as the bones of the spine weaken and collapse due to lack of calcium.

thyroid-function test looks at your overall metabolic rate. Parathyroid function and vitamin D metabolite tests indicate how stable your calcium levels are. Also measured is the level of osteocalcin, a blood component that provides information on bone formation. Another important role of blood testing is to rule out lymphoma, malignant myeloma (cancer of the bone marrow), and other malignancies that may be causing osteoporosis symptoms.

Urine is tested for calcium content and for two components associated with bone resorption: hydroxyproline and pyridinolines. Generally, if the calcium content in your urine is too low, it means you are absorbing calcium from your diet less effectively, while a calcium content that is too high is often a sign that the calcium is being robbed more rapidly from your skeleton. Abnormally high levels of hydroxyproline and pyridinolines in a urine sample suggest that you are losing bone density too rapidly.

Once you are under a doctor's care for osteoporosis, you will probably undergo blood and urine tests periodically to monitor the effects of treatment. According to the National Osteoporosis Foundation, blood and urine tests cannot detect low bone mass, however.

Bone density test

Regular X-rays can detect fractures, but they cannot detect osteoporosis until the process has advanced to the point where 25 to 40 percent of bone mass is gone, according to NOF literature. By then the patient's osteoporosis is so advanced that she can only marginally benefit from treatment.

To fill the detection gap, scientists and engineers developed a variety of highly sensitive techniques to measure bone density. These techniques—known as "absorptiometry" or "densitometry"—are considered safe, painless, and quite accurate. Although these bone-density measuring techniques vary, all are based on the same basic principle: the absorption of ionizing radiation by bone, according to Charles H. Chesnut III, M.D., of the University of Washington Medical Center in Seattle. The denser the bone, he explains, the more radiation it will absorb and the less radiation it will allow to pass through to a radiation detector.

The bone-mass measurement is known as the bone's "areal density." By comparing the areal density to what's considered normal for your age and body build, your doctor should be able to predict your future risk for fracture. If your risk is above average, preventive therapy, including hormone replacement, may be prescribed. In this way bone-mass measuring technology can enable your doctor to keep you from reaching the fracture zone.

There are at least five different techniques used to measure bone density. According to Dr. Chesnut, the "current state of the art" for measuring bone mass at the hip, spine, wrist, and total skeleton is dual energy X-ray absorptiometry (DEXA). DEXA produces an image that is easy to read, takes eight to ten minutes for a scan, and uses minimal radiation—about one-sixth of a chest X-ray per scan, Dr. Chesnut points out. Its precision is 99 percent accurate. Similar information can be obtained from dual photon absorptiometry (DPA), he says, but a DPA takes thirty minutes and its precision is 97 to 98 percent. Other techniques are radiographic absorptiometry (RA), used to measure bone mass in the hand; single photon absorptiometry (SPA), which measures density of the wrist and heel bones; and quantitative computed tomography (QCT), which measures spinal bone density. According to the National Osteoporosis Foundation, the cost of these tests runs from about $75 (RA and SPA) to $250 (QCT) per scan. DEXA subjects the patient to the least radiation exposure, QCT to the most.

Bone biopsy

During a bone biopsy, a small piece of bone is removed from the iliac crest and analyzed in a laboratory. The major reasons to have a bone biopsy are to rule out other bone diseases, to measure bone turnover, and to evaluate response to therapy, especially in patients who are responding poorly to treatment. The bone biopsy is a simple procedure, but is painful, invasive, and expensive. Since absorptiometry and densitometry can detect osteoporosis without invading the body, bone biopsies play a limited role and are seldom used. When deemed necessary, the biopsy should only be performed by a specially trained physician and laboratory personnel.

MOST COMMON FRACTURE SITES

It can't be overemphasized that since losing bone density is a painless phenomenon, most people don't learn they have osteoporosis until they break a bone. Some women suspect they have osteoporosis when they notice the development of a hump in their upper back. Others simply begin to lose height but don't realize it; this manifestation of developing osteoporosis is known as "painless curvature of the spine."

Theoretically, osteoporosis can precipitate a fracture of almost any bone in the body. But certain bones are more vulnerable than others either because of their location or because of the ratio of trabecular to cortical bone. Flat bones, such as the vertebrae, are more prone to fractures because they contain a higher percentage of trabecular tissue. Trabecular tissue (the spongy interior) is lost faster in osteoporosis compared with the dense cortical bone.

For those with full-blown osteoporosis, the spine, hip, and wrist are the most common fracture sites. According to the

NOF, osteoporosis leads to more than 1.3 million bone fractures each year: more than 500,000 vetebral fractures, 300,000 hip fractures, 200,000 wrist fractures, and 300,000 fractures of other bones.

The spine

More than one-third of women over 65 have at least one vertebral fracture, also known as crush or compression fractures. Crush fractures may be caused by minor trauma or sudden movement or may happen over time under the pull of gravity. Women are seven times more likely than men to experience a crush fracture, with women between ages 55 and 75 at the greatest risk. Crush fractures can cause pain that is often debilitating. These fractures result in a loss of height and may eventually result in a humped back, known as "dowager's hump." Crush fractures also can produce scoliosis, a deformity in which the spine is bent toward one side, according to the AMA's *Encyclopedia of Medicine*.

Once a vertebra is crushed, nothing can be done to restore the vertebra to a normal state. Acute pain from a crush fracture can last several weeks or months, and pain stemming from spinal deformity can persist indefinitely. Analgesics, heat, massage, and possibly brief bed rest can often alleviate acute pain. Those with chronic back pain may benefit from gait training, instruction in proper posture, and exercises to strengthen the back and abdominal muscles. Some patients are helped by wearing a back brace. Like all osteoporosis sufferers, patients with vertebral fractures are urged to stay active, increase their calcium intake, and take steps to prevent falls.

Hip fracture

The longer you live, the greater your chances of fracturing your hip, with almost one-third of women and 17 percent of men sustaining a hip fracture by age 90. Studies show that women age 65 to 85 are at the greatest risk. Many doctors believe that in about half of hip-fracture cases, the osteoporosis-weakened hip breaks first, causing the patient to tumble to the floor. In the other half of cases, the hip breaks upon the impact of falling. According to the American Association of Retired People (AARP), most hip fractures occur in the home. A fractured hip leads to the inability to walk, which may or may not be permanent. To aid in healing, screws can be surgically implanted into the hip joint.

Wrist fracture

Wrist fractures, including Colles' fractures, are six times more common in women than in men. The most frequent cause of wrist fractures is falling at work or anywhere outside the home, according to the AARP. Wrist fractures should be treated with immobilization as soon as possible. Casting of the whole arm promotes rapid healing, usually in six weeks. It's important that the casting be done by an experienced physician since a badly done cast can aggravate the fracture and prolong the recovery period.

PART II
TREATING
OSTEOPOROSIS

CHAPTER 6

THE ESTROGEN CONNECTION AND OTHER DRUG THERAPIES

If ever there were a magic elixir to prevent osteoporosis, estrogen comes close. Estrogen has been shown to prevent the dramatic loss in bone density that occurs during the first five to eight years following menopause. Studies suggest estrogen can even prevent fractures in women with established osteoporosis. Estrogen, a female sex hormone, has other important health benefits, such as lowering the risk for heart disease by about 50 percent. Estrogen also alleviates hot flashes and other distressing menopausal symptoms.

But taking estrogen after menopause, a regimen known as hormone replacement therapy (HRT), is by no means a panacea. HRT has generated controversy in the medical community, which continues to debate its overall safety in the wake of conflicting research findings. Women who opt for HRT must be careful to comply with the prescribed treatment protocol and get checkups every six to twelve months. Estrogen must be taken regularly for several years in order to reap the bone-strengthening effect.

Estrogen replacement has been associated with a possible but unlikely elevated risk for breast cancer and a definite but small elevated risk for endometrial cancer. Estrogen can be prescribed with another hormone, progestin, which helps protect against endometrial cancer but may blunt estrogen's protective effect on the cardiovascular system. Only women who have had their uterus surgically removed should take estrogen alone.

Estrogen and progestin can trigger menstrual-like bleeding in postmenopausal women. Patients should also be aware that HRT does not protect them against stroke and does nothing to alleviate osteoporotic pain. In addition to possibly raising the cancer risk, potential side effects of estrogen therapy include headaches, weight gain, depression, high blood pressure, thrombosis (blood clot in a blood vessel), and gallbladder or liver disease. Fear of cancer and other possible adverse effects dissuade some women from taking HRT.

Why estrogen?

The relationship between loss of ovarian function and bone loss was first described in the early 1940s. It wasn't until this decade that scientists identified estrogen receptors on bone cells that are involved in remodeling. The discovery provided the strongest evidence to date that there is a direct connection between the loss of estrogen and the loss of bone, particularly trabecular bone.

It is thought that the loss of estrogen increases the number of resorption cavities in the skeleton. Experts believe that once estrogen therapy begins, these cavities begin to be filled and the activation of new resorption sites is probably slowed. As a result, bone turnover is reduced and density is preserved.

As mentioned earlier in this book, women lose up to 3 percent of their bone mass annually during the five to eight years immediately following menopause. As a result, more than half of all women will develop osteoporosis after their sixty-fifth birthday and some will already have fragile bones in their fifties. By contrast, bone loss in premenopausal women ages 35 and older is only about 1 percent a year.

What is menopause?

Menopause, sometimes called the "change of life," occurs when your ovaries produce so little estrogen that you cease producing eggs and having periods. The gradual shutdown of ovarian function, called "perimenopause," usually begins between ages 45 and 55 and lasts several months to a year, during which periods may be irregular until they stop completely.

Menopause and all of its ramifications, including bone thinning, also follow surgery to remove both ovaries from women of childbearing age. In addition to irregular periods, about 70 percent of menopausal women suffer hot flashes, which is the reddening of the face and neck accompanied by a sensation of heat, lasting a minute or two. Other symptoms often include night sweats, vaginal dryness, a frequent urge to urinate, and dry skin and scalp. Then there are the psychological symptoms, such as poor memory, inability to concentrate, tearfulness, anxiety, and loss of interest in sex, according to the AMA's *Encyclopedia of Medicine*.

The fact that menopause also leads to a reduction in bone density is mentioned in the encyclopedia's listing of menopause symptoms, but not until the end of the entry. Osteoporosis may not be the first thing most menopausal women think about when they are awakened by night sweats or struggle with marital problems because they no longer want to have sex. Postmenopausal bone thinning is not only invisible, it may not manifest in fractures for a decade or more. Only then will some women realize that they may have stepped onto the slippery slope toward more fractures, possible loss of independence in case of a hip fracture, or even death.

Despite the prevalence of osteoporosis and its potential dangers, the bone-protecting effect of estrogen therapy traditionally was viewed as a bonus of HRT. The primary reason most physicians recommended HRT for qualifying patients was to alleviate severe menopausal symptoms. Recently, doctors began recommending HRT to help protect patients against cardiovascular disease.

Even more recently has osteoporosis risk been figured into the equation. Obviously, reducing a woman's heart disease risk remains a strong argument for HRT. But HRT is now considered a "cornerstone of drug therapy for prevention and management of osteoporosis" in menopausal and postmenopausal women, according to Robert R. Recker, M.D., of the Center for Hard Tissue Research at Creighton University School of Medicine in Omaha, Nebraska. Studies have shown that taking HRT beginning at menopause prevents bone loss for at least ten to fifteen years (to age 75) as long as estrogen therapy is continued. Beginning HRT in the perimenopausal period—when periods become irregular but before they stop completely—may actually be most beneficial because some women begin losing bone at that time.

Even women who went through menopause years ago may be able to prevent osteoporosis by beginning HRT now. Writing in the *Journal of Clinical Endocrinology and Metabolism* in 1993, Dr. Recker notes that long-term HRT beginning more than six years after menopause will result in an overall bone gain of about 3 to 5 percent over a period of about twelve months. In the spine, estrogen increases bone mass by 8 to 10 percent, according to Robert Lindsay, M.D., Ph.D., of Helen Hayes Hospital in Haverstraw, New York.

Women who begin estrogen therapy a few years after menopause will enrich their skeleton, but they won't regain the peak bone mass they had at age 30. "If, on the other hand, estrogen intervention occurs early in the postmenopausal period," Dr. Lindsay writes in a 1993 edition of *Osteoporosis International,* "bone mass will be maintained at a value close to that achieved in the early part of adult life."

Most important, HRT prevents "all types" of osteoporotic fractures, "even for some years after it is discontinued," Dr. Recker writes. In a 1991 update published by the National Osteoporosis Foundation, Dr. Lindsay notes that hip and wrist fracture risks apparently are cut by about 50 percent in patients on HRT and vertebral crush fractures "may be reduced by as much as 60 to 80 percent."

He adds, however, that it is unclear how long a woman must take HRT to reap a meaningful reduction in fracture risk. "Early data suggested that at least five years of treatment would be required, but more recent data have suggested that reduction in hip fracture risk is seen only among women currently using estrogens and that past users retain little protection," Dr. Lindsay's report states.

Despite the benefits of estrogen, Dr. Recker says, it is estimated that no more than 10 to 15 percent of women who could benefit from HRT are receiving it at any point in time. Research has shown that up to 25 to 30 percent of estrogen prescriptions are never filled and about 50 percent of patients who begin HRT discontinue treatment within six months. Patients can be discouraged by the inconvenience of periodic bleeding, distressing mood swings, fear of uterine or breast cancer, and fear of stroke or hypertension, Dr. Recker explains.

Estrogen and breast cancer

Population studies of estrogen's effect on breast cancer risk have yielded some conflicting and confusing results. Several studies show that women on estrogen therapy for more than ten years run a small increase in breast cancer risk. Other studies "have failed to confirm any excess (breast cancer) risk associated with estrogen use." Whether the breast cancer risk is greater in long-term estrogen users or only in current users also is unclear, says Dr. Recker.

As a result of the inconsistent research findings, different physicians use different criteria for deciding which patients are HRT candidates. To play it safe, most physicians refuse to prescribe estrogen therapy for any patient who has a history of breast cancer or certain other breast diseases, such as recurrent benign cysts. Sarah Steele, a 62-year-old Florida resident with severe osteoporosis, underwent a mastectomy in 1977 and has since shown no signs of breast cancer recurrence. Nonetheless, she has been unable to find a doctor who will prescribe HRT for her, even though she is willing to assume the possibly elevated breast cancer risk.

If she had never had breast cancer, most doctors would probably offer her HRT with caveats: She must first have a thorough breast exam including mammography, which must show her breasts are healthy. Mammography screening must be repeated each year, whether or not her insurance covers the breast X-ray. Also, Sarah would have to be taught to conduct a breast self-exam and perform it diligently at least once a month, reporting any suspicious change to her doctor immediately.

Menopausal women who are undecided about HRT can request a bone-mass measurement (see Chapter 5) and a blood lipid (blood fats) test to assess their risk factors for osteoporosis and heart disease, respectively. Since every woman is different, physicians must counsel each patient, taking her individual situation into consideration before deciding whether to recommend HRT.

Estrogen and endometrial cancer

Women who still have their uterus raise their risk for endometrial cancer about four- to tenfold when they begin taking estrogen. This elevated risk can be greatly reduced by combining estrogen therapy with progestin. "Progestins do not interfere with the effects of estrogen on the skeleton, and it is possible that some progestins enhance the skeletal effects of estrogen," Dr. Lindsay writes in *Osteoporosis International*.

Who's a candidate for HRT?

No breast cancer history in your family does not mean your doctor will automatically put you on HRT just to prevent osteoporosis. Experts generally recommend HRT for white women whose ovaries were removed before age 50 and for women who had natural menopause but who have multiple osteoporosis risk factors, such as early menopause, bone density below normal for her age, or a blood relative with osteoporosis. The NOF stresses that, considering the potential side effects, the decision to take HRT should be made only after a comprehensive discussion with your doctor.

How estrogen is administered

If you decide to take HRT, you have another choice to make. Estrogen can be administered orally, through a skin patch, or vaginally. Estrogen seems to be most effective against osteoporosis when taken orally or through the skin patch. To minimize estrogen's potentially harmful effects, the current trend is to administer a relatively low dose, which produces a blood concentration of estrogen that is about equal to what the body produced naturally prior to menopause. Taking too low a dose may not be protective against osteoporosis.

There are multiple HRT regimens that doctors prescribe and which one is best for you depends on your circumstances. If you are on a cyclical regimen, you may experience a few days of light menstrual bleeding before the next cycle begins. If you spot or have excessive bleeding between periods, report this to your physician, who may order a diagnostic D & C (Dilatation and Curettage). Cyclical bleeding usually subsides after six months of HRT. Taking progestin continuously with the estrogen will prevent periodic bleeding. If the uterus has been surgically removed, estrogen is given every day without progestin.

No treatment is an island

HRT and the other osteoporosis treatments described below work best when combined with adequate calcium intake and exercise. Some investigators believe that estrogen's protective effect on bones may be enhanced by ingesting at least 1,000 mg of calcium daily. Calcium and other nutritional factors and exercise will be explored in subsequent chapters.

CALCITONIN

If you cannot take estrogen for any reason, there is one other approved medicinal therapy that can help you: calcitonin.

Discovered thirty years ago, calcitonin is a type of hormone made by the thyroid gland. Doctors realized that calcitonin was able to reduce bone turnover by suppressing the activity of osteoblasts, the cells responsible for bone resorption. For use as a drug, calcitonin is synthesized in the lab and resembles the naturally occurring salmon and/or human compound. The reason salmon calcitonin is favored is that its potency is greater and it has a longer-lasting effect in the human body.

In some studies, calcitonin has been shown to increase bone mass modestly. The main goal of osteoporosis treatment at this time, however, is to prevent further loss of bone, and calcitonin has been clearly demonstrated to do that. One study found that bone mineral in the spine increased up to 8.5 percent in one year of treatment with 100 IU (international units) of salmon calcitonin daily. Subjects who took the same dose of salmon calcitonin every other day for a year had only a 4 percent rise in bone density.

While it seems logical to assume that any rise in bone mass will lead to a lower risk for fractures, no studies have explored whether calcitonin therapy does, in fact, prevent fractures or reduce patients' risk for fractures.

In addition to treating postmenopausal osteoporosis, salmon calcitonin may be an appropriate treatment for people who develop secondary osteoporosis from overexposure to corticosteroids as a result of Cushing's disease or long-term steroid therapy (see Chapter 3). Salmon calcitonin can be administered along with corticosteroid therapy to prevent bone loss in the first place. This treatment has not been established as a preventive therapy, but many physicians have been using it with success. Men with age-related osteoporosis may also benefit from salmon calcitonin.

The most visible and immediate benefit of calcitonin is that it can alleviate the sometimes excruciating pain caused by osteoporotic fractures. This analgesic effect increases patients' mobility. Some doctors use it to treat the pain of an acute compression fracture. Relief usually occurs after a week or two of treatment.

Salmon calcitonin comes in two forms: injectable and nasal spray, but only the injectable form is currently approved in the United States for treatment of osteoporosis. In Europe, intranasal salmon calcitonin has proven safe and effective in preventing further bone thinning. It is used abroad also as an alternative to hormone-replacement therapy to prevent postmenopausal bone loss. When taken intranasally, salmon calcitonin appears to provide more effective pain relief and has fewer adverse side effects than the injectable form. About 5 to 10 percent of salmon-calcitonin users may experience urinary frequency, flushing of the face and hands, abdominal fullness, nausea, and skin rash.

Taking the drug just before going to bed can often minimize these effects. Other ways to reduce side effects is to take calcitonin a few hours after eating and begin treatment at a low dose and gradually increase the dose until it reaches an effective level.

The cost of injectable salmon calcitonin is about $1,000 to $1,500 a year. U.S. Food and Drug Administration approval is anticipated for the nasal-spray version in the not too distant future. Meanwhile, studies are under way to test the safety and effectiveness of giving salmon calcitonin orally, rectally, through a skin patch, and via implanted pump.

EXPERIMENTAL DRUG THERAPIES

Bisphosphonates

Bisphosphonates are chemical compounds that were originally used to soften hard water to prevent bathtub ring. They have been used to treat osteoporosis on an experimental basis only.

The ability of one bisphosphonate, etidronate, to cure a child of a rare bone disease was discovered accidentally many years ago. Etidronate and pamidronate are the only bisphosphonates approved by the FDA for treatment of Paget's disease of bone and other bone disorders but not for osteoporosis. Bisphosphonates appear promising in their ability to prevent bone loss and build bone density among osteoporosis patients, however.

Several hundred osteoporosis patients in the United States and Europe experienced an increase in bone density and a decrease in fractures after taking bisphosphonates on an experimental basis. According to an article in the July-August 1993 issue of the *Cleveland Clinic Journal of Medicine,* etidronate or pamidronate increased bone density from 1.2 to 7.8 percent a

year in postmenopausal osteoporotic women. Overall, etidronate (sold under the brand name Didronel) is a very well-tolerated
drug, which only needs to be taken two weeks out of every three
months. Possible side effects include gastrointestinal symptoms,
such as diarrhea, bloating, and spasms. Taking bisphosphonates
on an empty stomach may reduce these symptoms.

Researchers are hopeful that further studies will result in
FDA approval of bisphosphonates to treat osteoporosis. That
approval is unlikely to occur before the end of this decade, however.

Sodium fluoride

Everyone knows that fluoride salts help make teeth harder
and more resistant to cavities. That's why many municipalities
fluoridate their water supplies and many dentists give their
young patients fluoridated mouth rinses. Teeth are similar to
skeletal bone, so in the early 1960s experimenters decided to
give fluoride to people with osteoporosis. Since then a number
of other studies have looked at fluoride's effect on osteoporosis—with curious results.

For example, sodium fluoride produces a 5 to 10 percent
increase in spinal bone density for up to four years in many osteoporosis patients, David M. Slovik, M.D., of Harvard Medical
School, told doctors who attended an osteoporosis conference in
the spring of 1993. But the increase was confined to trabecular
bone. Cortical bone density continued to decline. These findings, Dr. Slovik says, suggest that sodium fluoride spurs a redis-
tribution of calcium within the body.

More worrisome is a large study that documented a three-
fold increase in the number of nonspinal fractures among osteoporosis patients who took 75 mg of sodium fluoride a day. And
Dr. Slovik points out that even though fluoride therapy increased spinal bone density in these patients, it failed to reduce

their rate of vertebral crush fractures. These findings suggest that fluoride therapy makes bones thicker but more brittle. There are no data on the long-term effects of fluoride therapy.

Combining fluoride with calcium, however, appears to combat osteoporosis without severe adverse side effects. As part of an ongoing research study, investigators at the University of Texas Southwestern Medical Center demonstrated that postmenopausal osteoporotic women who took fluoride and calcium citrate in a carefully controlled regimen were able to decrease the number of new spinal fractures by 50 percent and increase bone mass in the spine by about 5 percent a year. "Intermittent slow-release sodium fluoride plus continuous calcium citrate, administered for about 2.5 years, inhibits new vertebral fractures, increases the mean spinal bone mass . . . , and is safe to use," concluded the researchers, whose study was published in the April 15, 1994 issue of *Annals of Internal Medicine.*

Specifically, the regimen calls for taking 25 mg of slow-release sodium fluoride twice daily in repeated fourteen-month cycles (twelve months on treatment followed by two months off), and 400 mg of calcium citrate twice daily continuously.

Earlier studies showed that about half of the patients who have taken sodium fluoride therapy alone suffered adverse side effects, such as nausea; vomiting; pain in the feet, ankles, and knees. Lower doses of sodium fluoride may produce fewer side effects, Dr. Slovik suggests.

Other potential therapies

Echistatin, a component of snake venom, has been found to inhibit bone resorption. Much more research is needed to determine whether echistatin is a viable therapy for osteoporosis, however.

Diuretics, specifically thiazide diuretics, have reduced both bone loss and fractures in some patients who have taken the drug experimentally to treat their osteoporosis. But in the absence of large-scale studies, diuretics' role in osteoporosis prevention or treatment is unclear. Thiazide diuretics are mostly used in settings where more potent drugs can't be used because of their cost or because patients cannot tolerate other treatments. Diuretics have several untoward side effects that limit their usefulness, such as electrolyte imbalances and changes in blood lipid levels.

Tamoxifen, a man-made compound, is frequently given to breast cancer patients. Laboratory and animal studies suggest that tamoxifen has a bone-protecting effect similar to estrogen's. One study of postmenopausal breast cancer patients found that the bone density in their lumbar spine increased by 0.61 percent a year after taking tamoxifen. By comparison, breast cancer patients who took no tamoxifen lost about 1 percent of bone from their spine each year. As with estrogen, some recent studies have demonstrated increased risk of cancer with tamoxifen.

CHAPTER 7

THE NUTRITION CONNECTION

When you were born, your skeleton contained approximately 25 grams of calcium. At age 30 to 35, when your bone density reached its peak, your skeleton harbored about 1,000 grams—about 2.5 pounds—of calcium. The only means of gaining all that calcium is through your diet. But how much calcium should you take in each day to help maintain bone strength? What if you can't digest dairy products, the richest source of dietary calcium? Are all calcium supplements alike? Are there ways to up your calcium intake without drastically altering your diet? Is calcium the only nutrient you need to reinforce your bones? This chapter addresses these and other questions about nutritional influences on osteoporosis.

CALCIUM: THE SKELETON'S BEST FRIEND

Calcium, the body's most abundant mineral, plays several vital roles. It enables cells to communicate, muscles to contract, and nerve impulses to be transmitted from nerve endings to muscle fibers, and it helps blood to clot, according to the AMA's *Encyclopedia of Medicine.* In the skeleton, calcium combines with phosphorus to form calcium phosphate. This compound helps to make bones and teeth hard.

Before calcium can do its important work in the body, it

must first be absorbed through the digestive tract. People vary in the amount of calcium they are able to absorb from their diet, and absorption rates change throughout a person's lifetime. No one absorbs 100 percent of the calcium she ingests. Generally, healthy adults absorb only about one-third of the calcium they take in; the rest is excreted through urine and feces. Dietary fiber tends to reduce the amount of calcium that can be absorbed, and protein tends to increase the amount of calcium excreted in the urine.

Your body's ability to absorb calcium is at its peak during infancy. Babies absorb 67 percent of the calcium contained in human milk compared with 25 percent in cow's milk, according to the book *Breastfeeding and Human Lactation,* by Jan Riordan and Kathleen G. Auerbach (Jones and Bartlett, 1993). In the elderly, the intestine is less efficient at absorbing calcium. Heredity; certain drugs, foods, and diseases; and heavy alcohol consumption and smoking can all lower calcium absorption rates, as can insufficient levels of vitamin D. Limiting your coffee and tea intake to one or two cups a day and avoiding chocolate and caffeinated soft drinks may help you to retain more calcium since caffeine increases the amount of calcium excreted in the urine.

You also lose calcium when you sweat and shed skin, nails, and hair, says the National Osteoporosis Foundation. "That lost calcium is normally replaced from the calcium contained in the diet," NOF literature states. "When the diet does not contain enough calcium to offset these losses, the body breaks down bone in order to scavenge its calcium."

Moreover, a high-calcium diet appears to slow all age-related bone loss, except the bone loss that happens during the first five or so years after menopause. Researchers looking at communities with naturally occurring high calcium concentrations in their diet found a much lower instance of hip fractures as compared with communities with lower amounts of calcium in their food supplies. Naturally high calcium levels usually stem from water supplies. For decades, many communities have been adding fluoride to their water supplies to lower the incidence of dental cavities, particularly in children. If communities can fortify their water with fluoride, why not do it with calcium to help reduce osteoporosis?

One study published in the September 27, 1990, *New England Journal of Medicine* looked at 301 healthy post-menopausal women with a daily calcium intake of less than 400 mg. Half of the group increased their daily intake to 800 mg and "significantly" reduced bone loss, observed the study's authors, Bess Dawson-Hughes, M.D., and her colleagues at the U.S. Department of Agriculture Human Nutrition Research Center on Aging at Tufts University.

A life-long high-calcium diet also appears to reduce fractures. Several studies have found that the hip-fracture rate is reduced from 40 to 70 percent among people on a high-calcium diet. Another study showed that calcium and vitamin D supplementation reduced hip fractures in institutionalized elderly by 43 percent.

Of course, getting sufficient calcium in your diet won't by itself guarantee good bone health. Calcium is only marginally helpful against bone thinning spurred by immobilization or the withdrawal of estrogen, for example.

How much calcium is enough?

How much calcium you need each day varies according to your age, sex, and pregnancy status. Generally, calcium requirements are highest during adolescence and after menopause. Postmenopausal women on hormone-replacement therapy don't need as much calcium as their peers who are not on HRT.

Up to about age 10, the skeleton needs about 100 mg of

calcium per day, according to calcium researcher Dr. Heaney. That translates to an average dietary requirement of 500 to 600 mg a day, although the Recommended Daily Allowance (RDA) is 800 mg a day to allow for individual differences among children, Dr. Heaney says. U.S. government surveys show that most children are meeting that goal.

From adolescence through age 24, the RDA for calcium is 1,200 mg. Some experts believe that it should be about 1,600 mg for adolescents because people in that age group need more than twice as much calcium as they needed in childhood for proper skeletal growth.

Ruth Lufkin, Eastern Division administrator for La Leche League International, a breastfeeding organization, says that pregnant and lactating women probably need about 1,400 mg of calcium a day. Both the NOF and the National Institutes of Health recommend a daily calcium intake of 1,000 mg for premenopausal women and postmenopausal women on HRT. The calcium requirement is lower for these populations because female hormones improve calcium absorption and reduce calcium loss through the kidney, according to NOF literature. Postmenopausal women not taking estrogen and anyone at high risk for osteoporosis should get about 1,500 mg of calcium a day. The RDA for adult men is 1,000 mg.

At first glance, those large numbers seem like an awful lot of calcium. But you can get 1,000 mg by drinking three eight-ounce glasses of skim milk over the course of a day. Drink that much milk and add an ounce of Cheddar cheese and a sardine sandwich or a cup of plain, nonfat yogurt, and you've ingested 1,500 mg of calcium. Dairy foods provide about 75 percent of the calcium in the American food supply, according to the National Dairy Council. Vegetables containing calcium include turnip greens, broccoli, okra, and beet greens. Almonds, molasses, and canned fish with bones are other rich calcium sources.

Some food manufacturers have begun adding calcium to noncalcium-containing foods and adding more calcium to calcium-containing foods. Among other foods, calcium fortification can be found in certain brands of yogurt, orange juice, tofu, bread, soft drinks, milk, fruit punch, and cereal.

You can fortify your home-cooked meals by adding vinegar when making chicken soup (vinegar helps draw out calcium from chicken bones) or by substituting low-fat powdered milk for flour when making gravies. The Dairy Council recommends these other simple ways of upping your calcium intake: Make hot cereal or cocoa with milk instead of water, fill a melon half with cottage cheese or frozen yogurt, and add grated cheese to your salad, baked potato, or casserole. Calcium is best absorbed in a diet rich in complex carbohydrates, which are found in whole grains, pasta, vegetables, and fruits.

Despite the relative ease in getting enough calcium, a study entitled "Health and Nutrition Examination Surveys" (HANES) found that the average American woman takes in about 500 mg of calcium a day—only about half of what she needs. HANES also found that one in four postmenopausal women gets less than 300 mg a day. More than half of adolescent girls were getting less than 800 mg a day, far below the recommended daily requirement of 1,200 mg.

One reason so few girls and women get the calcium they need may be an obsession with their weight. As mentioned earlier, dairy products are the most plentiful source of calcium in the United States. Dairy products traditionally have been associated with fat. Fortunately, food scientists have figured out ways to remove most or all of the fat from virtually every dairy product from ice cream to cottage cheese. Stripping fat from dairy products does not reduce the calcium content. In some cases, such as milk, removing fat actually results in a product with more calcium than it started out with.

Another reason for a calcium-poor diet may be too much junk food. Snacking on potato chips is more appealing to the typical teenager than downing a cup of low-fat yogurt or cottage cheese. "The major problems in teen-age nutrition are that kids have money and access to inexpensive foods that offer poor nutrition," Fernando Cassorla, M.D., clinical director of the Institute of Child Health and Human Development of the National Institutes of Health, told *The New York Times Magazine* (October 3, 1993). "There's also peer pressure to eat fast food."

Another reason some people fail to get enough calcium is lactose intolerance. An estimated 40 million Americans are unable to digest milk sugars (lactose) because their small intestine doesn't have enough lactase, the enzyme that breaks down lactose. Lactose intolerance can be a lifelong problem or it can develop as you age. Symptoms of lactose intolerance include cramping, bloating, gas, and diarrhea after consuming milk or milk products.

In recent years, most drugstores have begun selling lactase drops and tablets that enable lactose-intolerant people to digest dairy foods. Two of these products are Lactaid and Lactrase, which are designed to be added to milk. There are also enzyme tablets you can take directly so that you can eat dairy foods anytime you want.

Most grocery stores, meanwhile, sell lactose-reduced milk as well as other dairy items already treated with lactase. These products taste sweeter than their nontreated counterparts. Other ways to cope with lactose intolerance is by consuming dairy products in smaller servings; drinking milk with a snack or meal; eating heated dairy foods, such as cream soup, custard, and pudding; and choosing yogurt, milk, or buttermilk with live acidophilus cultures, which help to break down lactose in the gut.

Calcium Content of Selected Foods

Food	Calcium (mg)
DAIRY	
Yogurt	
Plain, nonfat (1 cup)	452
Plain, low-fat (1 cup)	415
Fruit-flavored, low-fat (1 cup)	343
Milk	
Milk, skim (1 cup)	302
Milk, 1% low-fat (1 cup)	300
Milk, 2% low-fat (1 cup)	297
Milk, whole (1 cup)	291
Buttermilk (1 cup)	285
Nonfat powdered milk (¼ cup)	377
Chocolate milk, 2% (1 cup)	284
Malted milk (1 cup)	347
Cream half-and-half (1 tablespoon)	16
Light cream (1 tablespoon)	14
Cheese	
American, processed (1 ounce)	174
Bleu (1 ounce)	150
Brick (1 ounce)	191

Food	Calcium (mg)
Cheddar (1 ounce)	204
Colby (1 ounce)	194
Cottage cheese, creamed (1 cup)	126
Cottage cheese, 2% low-fat (½ cup)	77
Cream cheese (2 tablespoons)	23
Mozzarella, part skim (1 ounce)	183
Muenster (1 ounce)	203
Parmesan, grated (1 tablespoon)	69
Ricotta, part skim (½ cup)	337
Swiss (1 ounce)	272
Soups (canned, made with milk)	
Cream of chicken (1 cup)	180
Cream of mushroom (1 cup)	178
Cream of tomato (1 cup)	159
Desserts	
Baked custard (½ cup)	148
Frozen yogurt, plain (½ cup)	89
Ice milk, soft-serve (½ cup)	137
Ice cream, soft-serve (½ cup)	118
Ice milk, hardened (½ cup)	88
Ice cream, hardened, 10% fat (½ cup)	88

Food	Calcium (mg)
Pudding, chocolate (from mix)	150
Sherbet (1 cup)	96

NONDAIRY

Vegetables

Asparagus, cooked (⅔ cup)	21
Beet greens, fresh, cooked (½ cup)	82
Broccoli, fresh, cooked (½ cup)	89
Broccoli, frozen, cooked (⅔ cup)	88
Brussels sprouts, cooked (6–8 medium)	32
Cabbage, cooked (⅗ cup)	44
Carrot, raw (1 large)	37
Collard greens, cooked (½ cup)	152
Green beans, cooked (1 cup)	62
Kidney beans, canned (⅖ cup)	29
Lima beans, canned (⅗ cup)	27
Mustard greens, cooked (½ cup)	138
Okra, frozen, cooked (½ cup)	88
Onion, raw (1 medium)	27
Rhubarb, cooked (½ cup)	174
Sauerkraut, canned (⅔ cup)	31

Food	Calcium (mg)
Spinach, fresh, cooked (½ cup)	122
Squash, winter (⅖ cup)	21
Sweet potato, baked (1 small)	40
Tomato, raw (1 small)	13
Turnip greens, cooked (⅔ cup)	184
Fruits	
Orange (1 medium)	56
Orange juice, canned (8 ounces)	22
Prunes, dried (10)	43
Strawberries, raw (1 cup)	21
Tangerine (1 medium)	12
Watermelon (1 cup)	13
MISCELLANEOUS	
Almonds (¼ cup)	94
Fudge, plain (1 ounce)	22
Milk chocolate bar (1 ounce)	55
Molasses, blackstrap (1 tablespoon)	116
Perch, baked (3 ounces)	117
Sardines, canned, with bones (3 ounces)	372
Salmon, canned, with bones (3 ounces)	203

Food	Calcium (mg)
Sugar, brown (1 tablespoon)	11
Tofu, with calcium sulfate (½ cup)	434
Tofu, no calcium sulfate (½ cup)	130
Waffle, homemade (7-inch round)	179
MEALS	
Chef's salad, no dressing (1½ cups)	235
Enchilada, cheese (1)	324
Lasagna (2½-inch square)	460
Macaroni and cheese, homemade (1 cup)	362
Pizza Hut Supreme Personal Pan Pizza	520
Quiche (⅛ pie)	224
Spaghetti with meatballs (1 cup)	124
Taco Bell taco (1)	80
Wendy's broccoli-cheese potato	100

Sources: National Dairy Council, National Osteoporosis Foundation, and *Bowes & Church's Food Values of Portions Commonly Used,* 14th edition (Philadelphia: J. B. Lippincott Co., 1985).

Calcium supplements

Once word spread that calcium was an important component in osteoporosis prevention, a dozen or more brands of calcium supplements hit the marketplace. But is popping calcium
pills a prudent way to meet your daily allowance of calcium? Yes

and no. Your skeleton doesn't care where you get your calcium from, as long as you get it. So if your calcium intake is chronically low, your doctor may recommend supplementation as a way to meet your daily requirement. However, woman does not live by calcium alone. Studies have shown that people on low-calcium diets are typically deficient in other nutrients, too, such as magnesium, phosphorus, and vitamin D, all of which are important to bone health.

The body needs more than forty different vitamins and minerals every day to function properly, and the best way to get these nutrients is to eat a variety of foods. When you take a calcium supplement, you're only getting a chemical compound containing calcium. When you eat a serving of steamed broccoli, you're getting calcium, vitamin A, vitamin C, and fiber, too. Most multivitamins contain little or no calcium.

Whether to take calcium supplements is a decision best arrived at in consultation with your doctor. Your doctor or a nutritionist can help you determine how much calcium you are getting through your diet. Or you can use the list in this chapter to make your own estimate. If you have osteoporosis or are at high risk for excessive bone loss, your doctor may recommend supplements to make sure that you meet your RDA. No one should attempt to meet her RDA through supplementation alone.

Once you decide you need to supplement your calcium intake, the choice then becomes which supplement to use. The number of calcium supplements commercially available is exhausting and confusing. Which supplement to take is a common question that patients ask their doctors.

Calcium supplements come in tablet, powder, and liquid form. Some supplements need a doctor's prescription, but most are available over the counter. Each type of supplement contains calcium in combination with one or more other substances to form a salt (not to be confused with table salt, which contains sodium). The reason is that the body is unable to absorb a supplement that is 100 percent pure calcium.

It's commonly believed that you can judge how well your stomach will absorb a calcium supplement by placing the tablet in warm water or vinegar and seeing if it dissolves completely in thirty minutes. A much better indicator of absorbability, or "bioavailability," is the amount of elemental calcium the supplement contains. When reading the label, look for the elemental calcium content. For most supplements, you will find a range of about 9 to 40 percent. If the label fails to disclose the percentage of elemental calcium, select another supplement. If a tablet has 300 mg of elemental calcium, you should take three or four a day if you're trying to get a total daily intake of 1,500 mg. If the supplement contains 500 mg of elemental calcium, you probably need to take just two a day.

Calcium carbonate, made from oyster shell, generally contains 40 percent elemental calcium. Dr. Dawson-Hughes and her colleagues at the USDA research center concluded that calcium citrate malate is even more effective than calcium carbonate in preventing bone loss in postmenopausal women. Tums, the popular stomach antacid, contains 500 mg of calcium carbonate (200 mg of elemental calcium) per tablet and is considered a safe way to supplement your calcium intake. Other calcium salts include calcium phosphate, calcium sulphate, calcium citrate, and calcium glubionate, which at about 6 percent elemental calcium offers the lowest concentration of calcium.

You should probably avoid dolomite since it may be contaminated with traces of cadmium, uranium, mercury, arsenic, and lead. In general, you should also avoid calcium glubionate and calcium lactate because the amount of elemental calcium found in those compounds tends to be very low, but always read the label to be sure.

Bonemeal, which is made from cattle and horse bones, came under fire in the early eighties after a *Consumer Reports* investigation found that supplements made of bonemeal contained unacceptably high levels of lead. The lead could be traced to environmental pollution, which tainted the vegetation the animals ate. "The U.S. Food and Drug Administration . . . pressed the companies marketing bone meal to eliminate the problem," states an article in the October 1993 issue of *Consumer Reports*. Since then lead concentrations in bonemeal products "have dropped enough to make the health threat negligible for most adults," the article says. The magazine credited the phasing out of leaded gasoline and tighter FDA limits on the amount of lead in bonemeal.

"Bone meal is now not very different from other calcium supplements in terms of lead levels," the article continues. "Surprisingly, all types of calcium supplements can contain traces of lead, largely from natural sources." This is another reason to use supplements in moderation and only when your dietary intake falls short, the magazine advises.

Taking any calcium supplement with a vitamin C–containing beverage, such as orange juice or grapefruit juice, or with milk or yogurt helps the body absorb calcium more readily. Generally, though, it is better to take the supplement on an empty stomach, between meals, or just before bedtime. Do not take more than 500 mg of calcium at one time.

People prone to kidney stones should be particularly careful about taking calcium supplements or maintaining a high-calcium diet because calcium may aggravate the condition. Be sure to tell your doctor whether you've ever had kidney stones.

Calcium and healing

Getting adequate calcium and vitamin D as well as enough calories is particularly important while healing from a bone fracture. Studies have shown a 10 percent skeletonwide bone loss following fractures of the long bones "even in the face of 'adequate' calcium intake," states the medical textbook *Osteoporosis: Etiology, Diagnosis, and Management.*

Calcium controversy

There is little argument that a generous intake of calcium contributes to enhanced bone mass from childhood through the midthirties and that people who get very little calcium may experience bone loss after age 35.

Less clear is how much calcium postmenopausal women should take in to maintain their bone density. Several studies have suggested that calcium isn't quite as effective as previously thought in maintaining spinal bone mass in older women. But there is some evidence suggesting that postmenopausal women who get generous amounts of calcium every day may be able to reduce their estrogen dose and still keep their bones strong.

During the first few years after menopause, calcium in the absence of HRT does not maintain bone mass. This observation led a lot of researchers to argue that women need not increase their calcium intake after the change of life. On the other hand, women on HRT who were given extra calcium developed stronger bones than did women who were on high-calcium diets or estrogen alone. So while calcium by itself won't treat established osteoporosis, it appears to enhance the effectiveness of any treatment regimen. Until further studies paint a clearer picture, experts will continue to recommend that all adults get at least 1,000 mg of calcium a day and people at risk for osteoporosis get at least 1,500 mg a day.

Vitamin D

While calcium is the most abundant mineral in the skeleton, it is not the only nutrient involved in building bone. Getting enough vitamin D through your diet and through exposure to sunshine enhances your body's ability to absorb calcium. Children who don't get enough vitamin D may develop rickets. The RDA for vitamin D during growth is 400 IU, twice the RDA for adults. Elderly people probably should get 400 to 800 IU of vitamin D requirements each day since their digestive systems are less efficient at absorbing calcium.

Don't worry if you don't get enough sun exposure during the winter since the body can store vitamin D in fat for later use. To find out how much vitamin D is in processed foods, read the label. Food labels should tell you how much vitamin D a serving has and what percentage of your daily requirement that represents. Consult your doctor before taking vitamin D supplements, the National Osteoporosis Foundation warns, because too much can be harmful. The RDA of 400 units in a multivitamin can be taken safely.

Other nutrients involved in bone development include vitamin K, zinc, manganese, copper, ascorbic acid, and protein. If you have osteoporosis, a typical supplement regimen may include up to 1,500 mg of calcium carbonate and 250 to 350 mg of magnesium daily. Taking a multivitamin can also help to ensure that you're getting enough nutrients.

CHAPTER 8

THE EXERCISE CONNECTION AND PHYSICAL THERAPY

When astronauts from the Gemini space missions returned to Earth, their doctors noticed something peculiar. The astronauts' bones had lost some density even though they started out in peak physical condition. Thinning bones have also been observed in people who were bedridden for several weeks or months.

Fortunately, both the astronauts and the bedridden subjects regained the lost bone after resuming normal physical activities. If lack of gravity and inactivity lead to bone loss, can weight-bearing exercise strengthen the skeleton enough to prevent osteoporotic fractures? Studies on healthy people have demonstrated that the higher an individual's activity level, the greater her average bone density. Studies have also shown that people who are physically active have more bone mass than sedentary people.

Mehrsheed Sinaki, M.D., of the Department of Physical Medicine and Rehabilitation at the Mayo Clinic in Rochester, Minnesota, believes that a proper exercise program may increase bone mass and muscle mass at any age. Moreover, Dr. Sinaki writes in the March 1989 issue of *Archives of Physical Medicine and Rehabilitation* that a high level of physical activity throughout, but especially early in, life can result in increased skeletal mass during the third to fourth decades of life. A large reservoir of bone mass at midlife may delay or prevent osteoporotic fractures later on.

Exercising even after osteoporosis sets in may be able to re-build bone mass. A Danish study of women age 50 to 73 with previous wrist fractures found that the women who engaged in carefully prescribed aerobic and isometric exercises for one hour twice weekly increased the mineral content of their lumbar spine by 3.5 percent. The control group that got no exercise experi-enced a 2.7 percent drop in bone mineral density. "Physical ex-ercise may prevent spinal osteoporosis," concluded the researchers from Frederiksborg County Hospital in Hillerod, Denmark.

Unfortunately, not all studies of exercise and osteoporosis have demonstrated a correlation. It may be that certain types of exercises are more beneficial than others when it comes to osteo-porosis, and those particular exercises have not been included in the research. Or it may be that the study subjects did not exercise properly or long enough. Many doctors believe that longer, more carefully controlled studies will eventually prove that exer-cise can build bone, or at least slow or halt bone loss, in osteopo-rosis patients. But these doctors are not waiting for such a study to be done. Based on current research data as well as on their intuitive sense, these doctors are already recommending exercise as part of the osteoporosis treatment strategy.

Making such recommendations in the absence of conclusive evidence has sound precedent. Doctors began extolling aerobic exercise as a means of lowering their patients' heart attack risk years before researchers were able to prove beyond a reasonable doubt that aerobic exercise is good for the heart. As a result of the doctors' leap of faith, countless lives were prolonged.

How exercise affects bone

If you measure bone density in the arms of a right-handed professional tennis player, you'll find that her bone mass is greater in her right arm than in her left. The reason may be electricity. When muscles or bones are stressed, tiny electrical currents are created. There is substantial evidence that these so-called bioelectric impulses stimulate osteoblasts to create new bone. As explained in Chapter 2, there is a net gain in bone mass whenever osteoblastic activity outpaces the bone-digesting activity of osteoclasts.

The price of convenience

The enormous scope of osteoporosis can in part be attributed to the conveniences of modern society. We are tempted by certain habits—caffeine, alcohol, and tobacco—that can aggravate bone loss. Our diets are much lower in calcium than our ancestors'.

In more primitive societies, bone density was much greater because people walked everywhere and labored physically to hunt and gather food. The advent of the remote control means you can zip through television stations without rising from your easy chair. Drive-up banking and fast-food restaurants allow you to cash a check and eat lunch without leaving your car. The more convenient life becomes, the less physically active we need to be.

This is especially true for older Americans, many of whom are far less active than they were in their youth. This inactivity may stem from a fear of falling or the fact that they are not as strong and agile as they used to be and have less endurance. Older people also tend to tire more easily.

If you give in to your impulse to hang up your tennis racket or jogging suit, figuring you are "too old" for these pursuits, you may aggravate the bone loss associated with osteoporosis Types I and II (hormonal and age-related, respectively). This does not imply that you should play tennis as hard and long as you did when you were 25. If you were active throughout most of your life, you can modify your exercise routine while keeping it vigorous enough to maintain a strong skeleton. Even if you were sedentary when you were younger, it's never too late to start exercising, so long as you start out slowly and increase the intensity very gradually.

Writing in the *Osteoporosis Report,* a publication of the NOF, in 1992, Gail P. Dalsky, Ph.D., cautions that exercise should not substitute for, or delay the use of, medically accepted therapies in the prevention and treatment of osteoporosis. Exercise, writes Dr. Dalsky, who is director of the Exercise Research and Bone Mass Measurement Labs at the University of Connecticut Osteoporosis Center, should be considered as "adjunctive therapy" in combination with other treatment, particularly when a patient's "trend toward bone loss is strong."

What kind of exercises are best?

A bone-strengthening exercise program should probably include both aerobic and strengthening exercises. A proper aerobic workout raises your heart rate from a resting rate of 60 to 70 beats per minute to around 120 beats per minute for at least twenty minutes. Aerobic dancing (low-impact), stair climbing, jogging, ballroom dancing, brisk walking (especially while wearing a weighted belt), and racquetball are some examples.

"Activities which are weight-bearing or impact-loading, such as stair-climbing or volleyball, are more likely to stimulate increases in bone mass than non-weight-bearing or weight-supported activities, such as swimming or cycling," says Dr. Dalsky.

Isometric exercises, such as working out on Nautilus equipment or lifting free weights, strengthen your muscles and tendons, although there is no direct evidence that such exercises make bones denser. However, "it is statistically true that individuals with higher muscle mass have less osteoporosis, and in experimental animals and (test-tube) studies, electrical activity (as is generated from muscle) promotes bone growth and healing," write Mary M. Vargo, M.D., and Lynn H. Gerber, M.D., of the Department of Rehabilitation Medicine at the NIH in the August 1993 *Bulletin on the Rheumatic Diseases* published by the Arthritis Foundation.

A recent study advocated Tai Chi Chuan, a martial art known for its flowing body movements, as a "safe alternative to more traditional exercises because it combines weight bearing with a lack of joint trauma," according to the *Bulletin* article. The study did not measure the effects of Tai Chi Chuan on bone mass, but there is little doubt that stronger muscles and tendons help to protect bones during a fall.

Performing low-impact aerobic and strengthening exercises at least three times a week should also improve your sense of balance, which helps you to avoid falling in the first place. If you can't lift heavy weights, compensate by lifting lighter weights but increase the number of repetitions.

Any form of exercise or weight lifting—be it free weights or Nautilus or similar exercise equipment—should be initiated under an expert's supervision and built up very gradually. This is particularly important if you have been diagnosed with osteoporosis or osteopenia. If you can afford it, ask your doctor to refer you to a physical therapist or physiatrist to instruct you on the proper way to exercise. Otherwise, read the literature about exercise distributed by the National Osteoporosis Foundation and the Arthritis Foundation (some suggested exercises appear at the end of this chapter).

Exercise for several sessions with one level of weight and graduate to slightly heavier weights only when your muscles are strong enough. Don't increase the weight too fast. A woman with osteoporosis who picks up weights that are too heavy for her can initiate a fracture.

Some people with advanced osteoporosis symptoms should probably avoid such activities as golf, bowling, sit-ups, and other exercises that involve stooping or flexing the back or shoulders. Like the inappropriate use of weights, such movements can precipitate vertebral fractures.

If you are over age 50 or have a medical condition, get clearance from your physician before embarking on any exercise program. Your doctor may refer you to a physical therapist or physiatrist who is qualified to prescribe exercise routines that are appropriate for you.

Anyone with a known heart condition or who is at risk for cardiac disease should undergo a cardiology evaluation before beginning an exercise program. You may be advised to take a stress test, during which your heart is monitored electronically while you walk on a treadmill or ride a stationary bicycle. The test aims to detect any abnormalities in your heart rhythm while your heart is working at peak capacity.

People's physical conditions, interests, and tolerance levels vary widely, so let an expert design an exercise program that's appropriate for you. The program should be balanced, using all of the major muscle groups. The most important factor is enjoyment. "The realities of patient preference and convenience must be considered," write Vargo and Gerber. "A lesser-impact activity that the patient enjoys is better for long-term compliance than the 'chore' that is quickly dropped."

Adopting a more physically active lifestyle need not be expensive. Perhaps there's a park with a jogging path near your home. Jogging or power walking (walking while holding 3- or 5-pound dumbbells in your hands) on a track or a dirt path is less traumatic on your joints compared to a sidewalk or a street. Some indoor shopping malls are open to walkers before business hours, which enables you to walk during inclement weather.

Many hospitals, colleges, and senior-citizen centers sponsor low-cost exercise classes for older women. Before enrolling in an exercise class, make sure that the instructor is certified to teach older adults who may have physical limitations.

If you opt to join a health club, you can gain access to a variety of high-tech exercise equipment for both aerobic and muscle-strengthening workouts. Look for a club with machines that are well maintained. Resistance in some exercise circuits is controlled by compressed air rather than weights. In either case, you should be able to control the resistance easily without having to bend down to pick up or adjust weights. Also be sure that exercise coaches are on hand to show you how to use each machine correctly. If the club offers aerobics classes, select a low-intensity workout and quit early if you become winded. If you keep at it, the workout will eventually get easier and more fun.

If you prefer to exercise in private, you can buy an exercise video recommended by your doctor or physical therapist. Do the video workout in a room without any throw rugs or loose electrical cords to prevent accidents and wear a good pair of sneakers. Free weights are relatively inexpensive to buy, or you can use cans of soup as substitute weights.

You may also wish to invest in a piece of exercise equipment for your home. A stair-climbing machine, treadmill, or cross-country ski machine all are good choices.

Be sure to drink plenty of water before, during, and after exercising, and avoid exercising in the heat of the day. If you jog or otherwise exercise outdoors, there's less air pollution in the early morning.

Here are some exercises designed to strengthen the spine, hip, and wrist bones, the areas most often affected by osteoporosis. The exercises appear in an article by exercise physiologist Christine Snow Harter, Ph.D., assistant professor and director of the Bone Research Lab at Oregon State University, Corvallis, Oregon, in the September-October 1992 *Osteoporosis Report*. Using both dynamic and isometric contractions of the muscles, the exercises were tested on more than 1,000 men and women ages 18 through 85, Dr. Harter says, and very few experienced pain or discomfort. If you are currently a nonexerciser, check with your doctor before trying these exercises.

Begin with only one set of each exercise, Harter says, and stop if you feel pain or discomfort. Don't do these exercises too fast, and rest at least thirty seconds between each set. "After the 'desired maximum' has been attained," Dr. Halter writes, "light weights may be added to the arms and legs to increase resistance." Once your body gets used to the exercise routine, the entire program should take no longer than thirty minutes. Dr. Halter recommends performing the exercises three to six times a week.

Pelvic lift

Position: Lie on your back, arms on the floor and hands next to hips, knees bent and slightly apart, feet flat on floor. Action: Begin by pressing your waist into the floor, then slowly lifting the vertebrae off the floor, starting with the lower back, then the middle, and finally the upper back. Hold lift for 10 seconds, pressing the buttocks together tightly, then roll down one vertebra at a time, starting with the upper back, then middle and lower back. Desired maximum: 3 sets of 8 each, with a 30-second rest between sets. Purposes: Builds strength in hip and low-back muscles.

Diagonal lift

Position: Lying on right side, right knee bent, resting the weight of the upper trunk on the right forearm. The left leg is extended back and the left arm is reaching forward as far as possible, chest and head rotated toward the floor. Action: Lift the head, chest, left arm and leg together, using the right arm to help press the chest up. Hold 10 seconds, then release. Desired maximum: 3 sets of 8 each, with a 30-second rest in between sets. **Purposes:** Strengthens all of the back muscles and muscles of shoulder and hip.

Chest lift I:

Lying prone (facedown), legs slightly apart, chin on the floor, hands next to hips with palms turned toward ceiling. **Action:** Slowly lift the head and chest off the floor as high as possible, pressing the palms toward the ceiling and keeping the feet and thighs on the floor. Hold for 5 seconds, then release. Desired maximum: 3 sets of 8, with a 30-second rest between sets. **Purposes:** Strengthen back, hip, and arm muscles.

Chest lift II:*

Position: As in Chest Lift I, but place the tops of hands so that they are resting on either side of the middle back. **Action:** Slowly lift elbows, chest, and head from the floor as high as possible, keeping the feet and thighs on the floor. Hold the arch for 5 seconds, then release. Desired maximum: 3 sets of 8, with a 30-second rest between sets. **Purposes:** Strengthen back and hip muscles.

Chest lift III:*

Position: Same as in Chest Lift I, but with hands behind the head. **Action:** Slowly lift the head and chest from the floor as high as possible, keeping the feet and thighs in contact with the floor. Hold for 5 seconds, then release. Desired maximum: 3 sets of 8, with a 30-second rest between sets. **Purposes:** Strengthen back and hip muscles.

---

*This is a progression of exercise sets. Begin with Chest Lift I; progress to Chest Life II after you are able to comfortably perform all three sets of eight exercises, and to Chest Lift III after you can comfortably perform Chest Lift II.

Leg and arm lift

Position: Lying prone, legs together, right arm stretched out on the floor over the head, left arm relaxed on the floor by the left hip. **Action:** Slowly lift the head, both arms, and left leg off the floor. Hold for 5 seconds, then release. Desired maximum: 3 sets of 8, with a 30-second rest between sets. **Purposes:** Strengthens back, hip, and arm muscles.

Isometric head press

Position: Sitting in an upright chair, hands placed on the back of the head (not on the neck) with fingers laced. **Action:** Resisting with hands, slowly press the head back against the hands while opening the elbows and looking toward the ceiling. Hold for 5 seconds. Desired maximum: 1 set of 8. **Purposes:** Strengthen the muscles of the neck and middle back region.

PHYSICAL THERAPY

Exercising is appropriate for the at-risk patient and those who have fully recovered from an osteoporotic fracture. After you break a bone, your immediate goals become pain relief and healing.

To recover from a vertebral crush fracture, you will probably spend a week or two in bed, lying on your back with a pillow under your knees to take the pressure off your spine, according to *Osteoporosis: Etiology, Diagnosis, and Management*. The medical text also advocates moderate massage of the back muscles and heat during the first few days. Your doctor may prescribe some pain-relief medication as well. Some patients need a cane or other assistive device during the recovery period or beyond.

Sometimes changes in the shape of the spine or stretched ligaments can result in chronic pain—pain that persists many weeks or months after the fracture has healed. You can help yourself by improving your posture, doing proper back-extension and abdominal-strengthening exercises, and wearing a back brace, the textbook advises.

While the crush fracture will heal in time, the deformity will remain. A single crushed vertebra will not result in dowager's hump. Several crushed vertebrae will, so your focus after healing becomes preventing future fractures.

Healing from a hip fracture is a bit more involved. Some patients need a hip-replacement operation. Others must use a wheelchair until the fracture is healed. Afterward, physical therapy can help some patients regain function.

Wrist fractures are usually treated with a cast that extends upward to cover most of the arm. When the cast is removed, a physical therapist can guide you through exercises that can help you regain function and strengthen your arm.

CHAPTER 9

OSTEOPOROSIS AND EMOTIONS

Like any chronic disease, osteoporosis can wreak havoc on a patient's psyche. All sufferers are affected differently, depending on the severity of their condition, their pain threshold, their sense of self-esteem and vanity, their propensity toward depression, and whether they have friends and family members who can help them. Osteoporosis is a disease of aging and is therefore a reminder that your days of youth are over. If osteoporosis follows a total hysterectomy, you will also be grappling with a changing sense of femininity.

Osteoporosis patients typically feel frail, and some refuse to leave their homes or exert themselves in any way for fear of breaking a hip and falling. Complaints of depression, anxiety, isolation, frustration, sadness, hopelessness, confusion, and despair are not unusual. Here are patients suffering not only from physical pain but also possibly facing disfigurement (dowager's hump) and temporary or permanent loss of independence. If osteoporosis is one of several medical problems, the sense of losing control over your life may be magnified.

Some women, particularly those who have had only one fracture or none at all, take osteoporosis in their stride. They derive satisfaction from knowing they are doing everything possible to help themselves. Others become overwhelmed with the treatment choices, particularly the decision of whether or not to take HRT. The very idea of having to take medication for years is enough to send some women into an emotional nosedive.

Women with advanced osteoporosis are more prone toward depression and loss of self-esteem. A pronounced dowager's hump—or even the beginning of one—can make patients cringe every time they look in the mirror. One 70-year-old patient agonized over the fact that her clothes no longer hung right on her body. Another patient with advanced osteoporosis cried when she remembered her grandmother, who had a severe hump in her back.

Medical science cannot reverse the anatomical or structural damage caused by osteoporosis. But there are things patients can do to feel better. They can understand that, in time, their pain will be greatly reduced or even gone as the broken bones knit. Painkilling medication and calcitonin can help relieve acute discomfort. Proper exercise can often alleviate chronic pain.

If you have a bent spine, speak with a fashion consultant to find clothes and accessories that de-emphasize your back while flattering other parts of your body. It may also help to change your hairstyle or makeup—or anything that makes you feel better and more confident about your appearance.

When you are severely depressed, it's easy to lose your motivation to get help or follow your treatment protocol. Antidepressants may be indicated if your depression is impeding your ability to perform daily tasks. Women who fight their way out of their depression may find themselves empowered to pursue treatment with more determination and vigor.

It also helps to talk to someone about your feelings. Find a close friend or relative, a caring physician, or a psychotherapist skilled in counseling people with osteoporosis. Consider joining or starting a support group for women with osteoporosis. Many newspapers carry listings of self-help groups on a regular basis. Or join the National Osteoporosis Foundation. The NOF will keep you updated on medical and political developments pertinent to your condition. The organization also provides tips on diet and exercise to make your bones stronger. Perhaps most important, NOF membership helps you to remember that you're not alone.

The upside is that many osteoporosis patients can return to an active life. The process of bouncing back from a fracture or a bout with chronic pain can be a slow one, so patience pays off.

CHAPTER 10

HELPING THE NEXT GENERATION PREVENT OSTEOPOROSIS

Throughout this book we have stressed that achieving and maintaining good bone health is a lifelong responsibility. Consuming enough calcium, getting adequate weight-bearing exercise, avoiding too much caffeine, alcohol, and sodium; and laying off tobacco from childhood on can greatly reduce a person's osteoporosis risk. The approach is quite similar to heart disease prevention: Nonsmokers who get enough exercise and maintain a low-fat diet have a longer life expectancy than people who don't adopt a healthful lifestyle until after suffering their first heart attack.

If your mother or father died of congestive heart failure, it becomes even more important for you to follow heart disease prevention strategies. As in heart disease, heredity appears to play an important role in osteoporosis. If you have osteoporosis or have learned that your bone density is below normal for your age—and it does not stem from any medications you are taking—your younger sisters, daughters, and granddaughters are likely to suffer a similar fate unless they do something about it now.

According to the National Osteoporosis Foundation, some experts believe that young women can increase their bone mass by as much as 20 percent—a critical factor in preventing osteoporosis. Although a number of promising treatments are available, or soon will be, preventing osteoporosis is always preferable to treating the condition.

Your first step in helping your younger relatives is to be frank. Be candid about your diagnosis and tell your loved ones that you are concerned about their osteoporosis risk. Becoming aware that osteoporosis runs in the family can be a powerful motivator to take steps to prevent it. Not only can your daughter learn how to reduce her risk of fractures, she may be able to help you avoid future fractures by using the suggestions in Chapter 3 to make your home safer, for example.

Knowing that osteoporosis runs in the family is also an important factor in deciding whether to take estrogen replacement therapy after menopause. Too often, women have had to guess at whether their mothers or grandmothers had osteoporosis. As discussed in Chapter 6, weighing the relative risks and benefits of estrogen replacement therapy is complicated enough. Providing definitive information regarding a family history of osteoporosis can only make your decision easier.

The decision to build the strongest, densest bones you are capable of building should, ideally, be made early in life. Tell your female relatives, even the young ones, that their most important bone-building years will continue until their late twenties or early thirties. By paying attention to their bone health early in life, they will ensure that their skeletons will have an easier time withstanding the bone loss that comes naturally with age.

Here are some more tips you can give to your loved ones:

1. *During childhood and adolescence, try to get at least the recommended daily allowance of 1,200 mg of calcium, if not more.*

A study by Pennsylvania State University researchers found significant increases in bone mass among a group of girls age 12 to 14 who consumed about 1,320 mg of calcium a day. The extra calcium came in the form of two tablets of calcium citrate malate daily—roughly equivalent to an additional glass of milk. The supplements were given to half of the 94 girls enrolled in the study. The other half took a placebo. After eighteen months bone density scans showed that the girls getting the real calcium supplements had 1.3 percent more bone mass than those who took the placebo. The study was published in the *Journal of the American Medical Association* (JAMA) in August 1993.

Another study found that calcium supplementation was ineffective in pubescent and postpubescent youngsters but was quite effective in enhancing bone mass in prepubescent children. The study involved forty-five pairs of identical twins age 6 to 14, where one twin received about 1,600 mg of calcium a day through food and supplements and the other twin got about 900 mg a day through food alone. Among the twenty-two twin pairs who were prepubertal throughout the three-year study, the children who took supplements had an average of 2.8 to 5 percent more bone than their sibling did at various skeletal sites. As the researchers, C. Conrad Johnston, Jr., M.D., and his colleagues at the Indiana School of Medicine, state in the July 9, 1992, *New England Journal of Medicine:* "If the gain persists, peak bone density should be increased and the risk of fracture reduced."

Commenting on the Pennsylvania State study, two nutritionists on the American Academy of Pediatrics' Committee on Nutrition told the *Philadelphia Inquirer* (August 18, 1993) that without forty or more years of follow-up study, it is impossible to know whether increased calcium intake during childhood and adolescence will actually prevent osteoporosis in the future. The reason is that too many variables may intervene, including the girls' diet as they grow older and whether they take estrogen after menopause, committee chairman William Klish, M.D., told the newspaper.

2. *To increase the possibility that a high-calcium diet in childhood will indeed lead to osteoporosis-resistant bones in the*

future, maintain a high-calcium diet throughout the teenage and adult years.

A study that followed 156 healthy female college students over five years found that bone mass continued to increase until 28.3 to 29.5 years of age. "Physical activity and dietary calcium intake both exert a positive effect on this bone gain," the researchers, Robert R. Recker, M.D., and his colleagues, write in the November 4, 1992 issue of *JAMA*. "Changes in lifestyle among college-aged women, involving relatively modest increases in physical activity and calcium intake, may significantly reduce the risk of osteoporosis late in life."

If you are concerned about the fat content in calcium-rich foods, such as cheese and ice cream, go for low-fat or nonfat versions. Calcium content of low-fat and nonfat dairy foods is often equal to or greater than their high-fat cousins. Also be aware that certain nondairy foods are good sources of dietary calcium. Roasted almonds, mackerel, canned salmon with bones, sardines, tofu, kale, spinach, and collard and turnip greens all offer a good supply of calcium. Or you can choose calcium-enriched bread, juice, and other products with added calcium.

And don't let lactose intolerance prevent you from getting enough milk products. Lactase pills are commercially available and lactose-reduced products are proliferating in the dairy case. Some lactose-intolerant people can digest milk products if they take small amounts throughout the day. Take calcium supplements only on days that your calcium intake falls short.

3. Make sure you get enough vitamin D. One way is to get about fifteen minutes of unprotected exposure to sunlight on your face, arms, and legs each day, weather permitting. But be sure not to overdo sun exposure, and avoid direct sun exposure completely if you have any precancerous skin lesions, lupus, or other disorders that can be aggravated by solar radiation.

Another way to get vitamin D is through dairy products and foods that are fortified with vitamin D.

4. *Make exercise a part of your life.* Learn to play bone-strengthening sports, such as volleyball, racquetball, and tennis, which you can easily carry into adulthood. Or take up aerobic dancing, jogging, or working out on exercise machines, such as the stair-climber. Exercising for twenty or thirty minutes at least three times a week should be a lifelong habit.

There also are less fun ways young people can be physically active: doing household chores, for example. Lifting garbage cans and mopping floors on a regular basis can boost a girl's bone density, according to a *Prevention* magazine report. Citing studies of older women, the article says that those women who had engaged in physical activity at least four times a week as teens and young adults had almost a quarter of the risk for fracturing their hip of women who were less active in their youth.

5. *But don't overdo exercise.* Anywhere from 30 to 50 percent of elite women athletes and professional dancers develop an estrogen deficiency, stop having periods, and therefore become susceptible to osteoporosis later in life.

6. *Don't smoke, and avoid ingesting excessive amounts of alcohol, caffeine, protein, and sodium.* All of these substances have a calcium-depleting effect on the skeleton.

7. *If you know that osteoporosis runs in your family, ask your doctor to order a bone-mineral scan sometime before the age of menopause.* Also consider requesting a scan if you fall into any of the high-risk categories, such as being thin and small-boned and fair-complected, or if you have had stomach surgery. By detecting bone thinning early, you can step up your calcium intake and exercise regimen in an effort to guard against osteoporosis.

8. *When you approach the age of menopause, begin thinking about hormone replacement therapy.* Ask your doctor whether

you are a candidate for HRT before menopause symptoms begin. Taking estrogen diligently during the perimenopausal period and continuing therapy for several years hence will help you to drastically reduce the bone loss that would ordinarily take place. Perimenopausal HRT may even increase your bone density.

CHAPTER 11

THREE WOMEN'S STORIES

People diagnosed with osteoporosis have a battle to wage, and for many it's filled with minefields of pain, disability, and emotional distress. But the human body has a remarkable ability to heal itself, given the right treatment and lifestyle changes.

Following are the stories of three women with osteoporosis, two of whom are enjoying positive outcomes and one who is still in the throes of trying to recover. We hope that these women's stories will inspire you and your loved ones to take whatever steps are necessary to combat or prevent osteoporosis.

JUDITH "JUDY" DORMAN

At age 53, Judith "Judy" Dorman outpaces most of her peers when it comes to physical activity. She downhill-skis in Colorado and Utah every winter. She water-skis near her Fort Lauderdale, Florida, home. She belongs to a health club, where she participates in aerobic dance classes. She works two jobs and takes care of her ailing mother. Judy was even considering taking up Rollerblading, also known as in-line skating, until she learned in mid-1993 that she has the bone density of an 87-year-old woman.

"I'm scared to death," Judy says six months after learning about her condition. "It made me modify my lifestyle. I'm more afraid, more hesitant about doing things. I very much wanted to take up in-line skating. Now I'm afraid to take the risk."

Judy has osteopenia, a condition of chronic bone thinning that threatens to push her into the fracture zone. Sadly, she has a front-row seat to the fracture zone because her mother has suffered for years with dowager's hump and excruciating back pain stemming from osteoporosis. Despite her mother's condition, Judy didn't consider herself at high risk for osteoporosis "because I thought I took after my father's side of the family."

Judy, a petite woman with red hair and fair skin, was a milk drinker all her life. She also loves cheese, butter, and other dairy products.

When she entered menopause in her early forties, Judy asked her gynecologist for hormone replacement therapy in order to prevent bone loss, but he refused to give it to her. Two or three years later she asked again for HRT. Again the doctor refused, even though Judy had no history of breast cancer.

Judy was shopping for another gynecologist, one with a more open-minded approach to HRT, when she picked up a newsletter at Cleveland Clinic–Florida, a medical facility where she took her mother for treatment several times a week. The newsletter announced that one of the clinic's physicians, Dr. Johna Lucas, was looking for healthy women to participate in an osteoporosis study. "I was familiar with what a lack of good, solid bone can do to you, having gone through it with my mother," Judy says. "I wanted to do something to help other women avoid it."

After being accepted into the study, Judy was given a specialized scan to measure her bone density. The density in her spine and hip was so low that she had to drop out of the study. Judy, who had "no symptoms whatsoever" of thinning bones, was shocked.

"So now instead of helping somebody else avoid osteoporosis," she says, "I'm just hoping and praying that the study will help me."

Fortunately, Judy is already being helped by becoming a patient of Dr. Lucas's. She was put on HRT immediately and told to take calcium supplements and increase her level of weight-bearing exercise.

Finding time to exercise has become increasingly difficult as her mother's condition has deteriorated and the demands of her jobs increased. So Judy, a divorcée who spends sixty hours a week managing a nonprofit private-business organization and sells real estate on weekends, improvises whenever she can. While talking on the telephone in her office, for instance, she'll stand, sometimes on one foot, instead of sit. She takes the stairs instead of the elevator in the twenty-eight-story building where she works full-time. At home, she makes a point to walk instead of drive to any appointment whenever distance and weather allow.

But the ache that recently developed in her hip is giving her second thoughts about continuing to pursue her passion: downhill skiing.

The specter of osteoporosis has also fed Judy's other passion: warning others about the potentially devastating consequences of fragile bones. Not only can osteoporosis impair the victim's lifestyle, it also takes a toll on the victim's family members and friends who become caregivers, Judy emphasizes. She has already spoken to a women's civic group she belongs to, urging fellow members to ask their doctors about preventing osteoporosis. Judy says her previous gynecologist is partly to blame for her current condition because he refused to put her on HRT. In her experience, female doctors generally seem more aware of osteoporosis than their male counterparts.

"There is such a need to create an awareness, not just among my own 53-year-old peers, but among women of all ages," she says. "Younger women are just totally unaware of the ravages of this disease and totally unaware that they, too, may become victims."

ANTOINETTE "ANN" COSENZA

In the late 1970s, Antoinette "Ann" Cosenza developed pain in her back. The pain got worse and worse and was particularly severe in the morning.

"When I woke up, I could not get out of bed," says Ann, 62, a recently retired secretary. "I could not take a shower, it hurt so much. I could not sit up and type at work; I used to lean back in my chair, almost lie in it."

For two or three years, Ann endured back pain. When she told doctors at her health maintenance organization about it, they ordered blood tests but no X-rays. "Nobody came up with an explanation for why my back hurt all the time," Ann says.

When she came home from work each day, all Ann could do was sit in a chair. "I could not stand up and clean vegetables; I could not walk; I could not do anything with this chronic pain in my back."

In 1980, Ann, a divorcée, was living alone in Albuquerque, New Mexico, when her pain became so severe that it woke her up with a start in the middle of the night. "I jumped out of bed and fell on my bottom," she recalls. "Then there was this pain that went right up through my back. It was horrible.

"I said to myself, 'Oh, my God, don't faint, don't panic.'"

It took Ann a good half hour to hoist herself back onto the bed from the floor. It took her another fifteen minutes to reach the telephone and call a friend. Later that morning Ann forced herself to drive to her doctor. "He lifted up my arm and checked to see if anything was broken," Ann recalls. "Then he said I was okay, sent me home, and told me to lie on my back for a week."

Ann followed that advice. A week later, with extreme difficulty, she managed to go back to work. Still reeling from intense back pain, Ann took what seemed to her like hours to get out of her car and straighten up each morning. She had to put her hand in the small of her back in order to support herself standing up. Even her teeth were becoming loose. After several days of torment, Ann went back to her doctor and insisted on getting her back X-rayed.

Looking at the X-ray film, the doctor could plainly see that two of her vertebrae were crushed. It was obvious that Ann had advanced osteoporosis. "He told me that once osteoporosis shows up in X-rays, it means there's a lot of bone loss," Ann says. The doctor's only advice was "Take some Tums."

Even though Ann had never heard of osteoporosis before, she knew at that moment that "I'd have to fight for myself."

She went to the library and read everything she could find about osteoporosis, which, back then, wasn't much. But she did learn that she had several risk factors. She had a small build and was always "very skinny." She was lactose intolerant and had therefore avoided milk products most of her life.

After undergoing a complete hysterectomy in 1977, Ann had been given estrogen therapy by her gynecologist, but she hadn't taken it for long. "I knew what estrogen did to me," says Ann, who had suffered severe premenstrual syndrome and fibroids in her uterus before her operation. Back then, low-dose estrogen was not available. The high dose had made her angry and depressed.

As time went on, Ann began hearing more and more about osteoporosis. She heard the topic discussed on a radio talk show. The first osteoporosis book came out, and articles about thinning bone began popping up in women's magazines. After learning of the connection between diet and bone health, Ann decided to consult a nutritionist.

"Why are you looking so sad and depressed?" the nutritionist, Robert Downs (not his real name), asked during her first consultation.

"Because I can't function," Ann told him. "I can't go to the mall, I can't stand by my sink, I can barely sit. I'm in pain every day. It takes a half hour for me to get out of bed."

"I can help you," Downs promised.

"If you can," Ann told him, "I'll give you a kiss!"

The nutritionist urged her to swim and walk every day. He gave her Fortical, a calcium and magnesium supplement with vitamins D and A, cod liver oil, and "a lot of other vitamins," Ann says. He also told her to eat lots of turkey and green vegetables and to avoid sugar, salt, and caffeine. Ann was never a smoker or a coffee drinker, but she had to give up her beloved chocolate—except for the occasional binge. She was further advised to drink lactose-reduced milk. "He also wanted me to get massages and do some yoga," she says.

When Ann started her swimming regimen, she couldn't swim the width of the pool in her condominium complex without becoming exhausted. Walking was also a chore. But the nutritionist had told her to push herself. "So I pushed," Ann says. "I huffed and puffed and said to myself, 'I'll keep doing it if it kills me.' "

Ann also joined a yoga class and started getting massages every week. After several weeks, the nutritionist told her to begin isometric exercises using a three-pound weight in each hand. That step was particularly challenging for Ann, who says, "When you have osteoporosis, everything feels heavy."

Within a few months, Ann could tell she was getting stronger. She could swim the length of her pool without getting winded. She could walk three to four miles at a stretch.

"Six months after I first visited the nutritionist, I woke up and had no pain," she says. "It was a miracle. I went back to the nutritionist and said, 'It looks like you get your kiss.' "

Ann stuck to her exercise routine and calcium supplements for a couple of years. Her efforts continued to pay off. A scan in 1991 showed that her bone density was normal for a woman of her age. Her periodontist, who had told her she'd need $7,000 worth of dental work to pull out and replace her loose teeth, told Ann she no longer needed the dental work.

Believing her osteoporosis was cured, Ann cut back on her calcium supplements, made less of an effort to get adequate calcium through her diet, stopped swimming, and reduced her walks from four to two miles.

"Since I started feeling good, I became lax," Ann admits. In 1993, a second bone scan revealed that Ann was back in the fracture zone. Her teeth became so loose again, Ann says, that "I couldn't even eat an apple.

"But now I'm starting back on my diet and exercise routine," she vows. "I guess it's human nature to stop treatment when you're feeling good. But I've learned the hard way that if you don't use it, you lose it. It's very important to keep your body moving."

LESLIE GRANT

Leslie Grant (not her real name) of Pompano, Florida, never used to notice women with dowager's hump. Now she notices these hunched-over ladies all the time because she has become one of them.

"It's very common," says Leslie, 79, who owned a restaurant with her husband before she retired. "My left side is bumpy, but I try to get used to it."

Leslie was born in Germany and immigrated to the United States when she was in her teens. She describes herself as heavy-boned, which does not fit the profile of the typical osteoporosis patient, who is small-boned. But there are other facets of Leslie's life that made her vulnerable to osteoporosis early on. She drank milk as a young child, but not as an adult. When she began menopause at age 54, no doctor advised her to take estrogen. She didn't do much exercising beyond walking.

So when she developed pain in her lower back during a vacation in 1989, her physician immediately suspected osteoporosis. X-rays of her spine showed multiple compression fractures.

"I was surprised," says Leslie. "And I was also frightened by the pain. I was in agony."

From that point it seemed as if the "slightest thing" would precipitate another crush fracture; one fracture landed her in bed for more than three months. "I was out of bed for about a week, barely walking with a walker, and just by turning around another fracture happened," she says. "I also suffered a fracture while cleaning myself after using the toilet. It's frightening."

Leslie took painkillers to get over the period immediately following each fracture. When she felt better, she began going to a rehabilitation unit of her local hospital, where she engaged in light exercise under the direction of a physical therapist. She continued to use a walker to help reduce the pressure on her spine. Her therapy included light massage and placing a moist heating pad on the painful areas of her back. Leslie also joined a water exercise class.

She began drinking milk every day and taking calcium supplements on days she couldn't get enough calcium through her diet. Her doctor prescribed salmon-calcitonin injections, beginning with three doses a week and working up to five.

As of November 1993, Leslie felt "pretty good" and hasn't had a new fracture in about a year.

"I really can walk much better," she says, "and I hope to stay that way."

APPENDIX I

150 Most Asked Questions About Menopause, by Ruth Jacobowitz. (Hearst, New York: 1993; $15)

Estrogen, by Lila Nachtigall, M.D., and Joan Heilman. (HarperCollins, New York: 1991; $9)

Women and Hormones: An Essential Guild to Being Female, by Alice MacMahon, R.N. (Family Publications, Maitland, Fla.: 1990; $9.95)

Osteoporosis: A Guide to Prevention and Treatment, by John Aloia. (Human Kinetics, Champaign, Ill.: 1989; $12.95)

Preventing Osteoporosis, by Kenneth H. Cooper, M.D., M.P.H. (Bantam Books, New York: 1989; $18.95)

Calcium and Common Sense, by Robert P. Heaney, M.D., and M. Janet Barger-Lux. (Doubleday, New York: 1988; $16.95) (Out of print, but may be available in libraries or used book stores.)

APPENDIX II

National Osteoporosis Foundation (NOF)
1150 17th Street, N.W.
Suite 500
Washington, D.C. 20036-4603
(202) 223-2226

Nonprofit organization providing advocacy, news, and education about osteoporosis and its treatment and prevention. Membership dues: $10 a year; members receive quarterly newsletter, sixty-page handbook, and educational brochures.

American Association of Retired Persons (AARP)
601 E Street, N.W.
Washington, D.C. 20049
(202) 434-2277

Nonprofit organization providing advocacy, information, and education on issues affecting older Americans. Membership dues: $8 a year.

GLOSSARY

Absorptiometry: A technique used to measure bone density, also known as densitometry; types of absorptiometry include dual energy X-ray absorptiometry (DEXA), dual photon absorptiometry (DPA), radiographic absorptiometry (RA), single photon absorptiometry (SPA), and quantitative computed tomography (QCT).

Aerobic exercise: A form of exercise that accelerates the heart rate, such as dancing and stair climbing.

Anorexia nervosa: An eating disorder in which the victim is so obsessed with being thin that she maintains a starvation diet; primarily afflicts teenage girls and young women; victims are particularly vulnerable to osteoporosis later in life.

Areal density: A person's bone-mass measurement.

Bioavailability: A medical term used to describe how much of a nutrient the body is able to absorb and use after it is ingested.

Bisphosphonates: Chemical compounds that have been shown in experiments to preserve bone density and reduce the fracture risk; not approved for osteoporosis in the United States.

Bone biopsy: A procedure in which a small sample of bone is removed and studied.

Bone collagen: A type of connective tissue found in bone.

Bone density: The thickness, or mass, of bone.

Bone density test: A specialized scan that measures how thick bone is at various parts of the skeleton and how close to normal that measurement is.

Bulimia: An eating disorder in which the victim goes on food binges and then purges what she ate by forcing herself to vomit or by abusing laxatives.

Calcium: The most abundant mineral in the human body; essential to building bone.

Calcium phosphate: A chemical compound primarily responsible for making bone and teeth hard.

Calcium salt: A compound that is found in calcium supplements, such as calcium carbonate and calcium citrate.

Calcium supplement: A nutritional supplement that contains bone-building calcium; taken by people who cannot get their minimum daily requirement of calcium through foods alone.

Cancellous bone: The spongelike interior of bone; also known as trabecular bone.

Colles' fracture: A fracture of the wrist bone.

Cortical bone: A compact type of bone that forms the hard outer shell of the skeleton.

Corticosteroids: A type of steroid medication that has been associated with bone loss.

Crush fracture: A fracture of the vertebrae that occurs when the bone becomes so weakened from osteoporosis that it collapses; also known as compression fracture.

Cushing's syndrome: A disease caused by overactive adrenal glands that pump too much cortisonelike chemicals into the bloodstream; may stem from prolonged use of corticosteroid drugs, enlargement of the adrenal glands, or a tumor in the pituitary; can result in osteoporosis.

Densitometry: *See* Absorptiometry.

Dowager's hump: A severe curvature of the upper back that can result from multiple crush fractures of the vertebrae.

Echistatin: A component of snake venom that has been found to inhibit bone loss on an experimental basis.

Elemental calcium: The only type of calcium in a calcium supplement that can be absorbed and used by the body.

Estrogen: A female sex hormone that, among many other things, helps keep the skeleton dense and strong.

Fracture zone: When bone thinning progresses to the point where fractures begin to occur.

Geriatrician: A physician whose specializes in diseases of aging.

Hormone replacement therapy (HRT): Giving estrogen and sometimes progestin to certain women who have undergone menopause or are going through menopause; among other things, HRT helps prevent postmenopausal bone loss.

Isometric exercise: A form of exercise, such as weight lifting, that strengthens the muscles but does not necessarily speed up the heart rate.

Lactase: An enzyme found in the digestive system that breaks down milk sugar, or lactose, enabling a person to digest dairy products; can be added to foods to aid digestion.

Lactose intolerance: A condition in which the stomach lacks the enzyme lactase, which is necessary to digest milk sugars.

Menopause: The time in a woman's life, usually between ages 45 and 55, when the amount of estrogen produced by her ovaries begins to diminish and her periods subside.

Occupational therapist: An allied health professional who retrains patients to perform daily activities with an emphasis on safety awareness.

Osteoblast: A specialized cell that lays down new bone.

Osteoclast: A specialized cell that dissolves, or resorbs, existing bone.

Osteopenia: A potentially reversible condition in which bone loses density but not enough to result in fractures.

Osteoporosis: A condition in which bone thins out to the point where it tends to fracture from slight trauma or everyday stress.

Perimenopausal: The period of time when a woman's supply of estrogen begins to withdraw until estrogen production ceases almost completely; the perimenopausal period usually lasts about a year.

Physiatrist: A medical doctor who prescribes and coordinates the rehabilitation effort, including identifying risk factors for fractures and prescribing exercises, orthotics, canes, and medications.

Physical therapist: An allied health professional who helps make the home and work environments ergonomically correct and instructs patients on an exercise program ("ergonomically correct" means that your furniture, appliances, and other surroundings put little or no stress on your body).

Postmenopausal: The time of life after estrogen production ceases.

Power walking: Walking briskly with weights attached to the ankles, carried in the hands, or both.

Premenopausal: A woman's childbearing years.

Primary osteoporosis: When osteoporosis stems from menopause or aging.

Remodeling: A biological function in which the skeleton continually breaks down existing bone and replaces it with new bone tissue.

Remodeling unit: A discrete, microscopic area of bone in which bone-dissolving and bone-forming cells do their work.

Resorption: The dissolving of bone tissue by specialized cells called osteoclasts.

Salmon calcitonin: A type of hormone treatment designed to help preserve existing bone; often given to women who cannot take hormone replacement therapy.

Scoliosis: A curvature of the spine.

Seasonal bone loss: The type of reversible bone thinning that occurs in winter months when people tend to get less vitamin D–building sunshine.

Secondary osteoporosis: When osteoporosis is a result of an underlying disease, surgical procedure, or a drug the patient is taking.

Senile osteoporosis: Osteoporosis that results from aging; also known as Type II osteoporosis; the type of osteoporosis that affects men.

Trabecular bone: The spongelike interior of bone; also known as cancellous bone.

Turner's syndrome: A treatable chromosomal abnormality in which girls fail to produce estrogen and therefore never mature through puberty.

Type I osteoporosis: Postmenopausal osteoporosis, which stems from the loss of estrogen.

Type II osteoporosis: Osteoporosis that results from aging; also known as senile osteoporosis.

Type III osteoporosis: Drug-induced osteoporosis.

Type IV osteoporosis: Osteoporosis that results from an underlying disease.

Uncoupling: What happens when bone-dissolving cells and bone-building cells fall out of equilibrium, leaving the skeleton vulnerable to bone loss.

Weight-bearing exercise: Type of physical activity that places stress on the skeleton, such as aerobic dance, volleyball, and jogging.

INDEX

ABOUT THE AUTHORS

DR. YVONNE R. SMALLWOOD SHERRER attended the University of Pittsburgh School of Medicine, and completed her internship, residency, and fellowship at Stanford University. She now works at the Cleveland Clinic in Ft. Lauderdale, Florida, where she has served as the chairman of the Department of Immunology/Rheumatology.

ROBIN K. LEVINSON is an award-winning health and science writer.

She is the co-author of *A Woman Doctor's Guide to Infertility*. She lives with her husband and daughter in Hamilton, New Jersey.